A STORY OF HORRIFIC PAIN AND GREAT HOPE

Trigeminal Neuralgia Exposed:
"Our Story"

COMPILED BY JUNE TOLAND STEPHENS

Trigeminal Neuralgia Exposed: "Our Story"
First Edition 2015
Compiled by June Toland Stephens
Copyright © 2015

ISBN: 978-0-692-56691-6

Cover Image by Cheryl Lynn Poppe.

Inquiries about purchasing this book can be directed to June Toland Stephens at *TNExposedOurStory@gmail.com*.

Disclaimers

All statements, views and opinions presented in this book are solely those of the individuals making those statements and do not represent The Facial Pain Research Foundation or any other organization that may be mentioned herein.

The individuals in the book are not doctors, and their statements should not be considered medical advice. Readers should consult their own personal physicians or health care providers for any advice, course of treatment, diagnosis or any other information relating to their medical condition.

Dedication

This book is dedicated to all who suffer with trigeminal neuralgia (TN) and/or other facial pain, to The Facial Pain Research Foundation, and to the following TN sufferers that shared their stories and experiences in this book.

Allison Ramirez	Wendy Meek
Amy Popovich	Wendy
Anne Plohr Rayhill	Chris J Nolze
Betina Bach Knudsen	Kim Stephens
Brian Malecha	Dennis Gannon
Lisa Malecha	Kathy
Cathy L. McKinnon	Michele
Christy M. Ritter	Kaleigh Roberts
Debbie Murphy	Suzanne Martin
Gladys M. Rhodes	Barbara McDowell
Jennifer Click	Alphonse Pellegrino
Kiley Burns	Rebecca Thorpe
Kristi Leeder	Jenny LeCompte
Stacie Winslow	Kimberly Marin
Manuela Bradshaw	Pam Whitling Elliott
Matthew Williams	Jane Harris Kelley
Melissa Waters	Dennis L Wiant
LeeAnn Ryan	Dianna L. DeMay
Mark Gaubert	Rebecca Webb
Pat Zadorozny	Sarah Edmondson
Patti	Connie Fini
Pauline Donye	Christine Stefanik-Spor
Sheri Neumoyer	Margaret L. Dennis, D.M.D.
Suzi Strand	Betsy Taylor Alexander

A Collective Effort

This project began as the vision of one woman, June Toland Stephens, who enlisted numerous TN sufferers to describe their experiences. The book was written via a Facebook support group. The pages of this book contain the collective picture of trigeminal neuralgia as experienced by more than 50 sufferers from around the world that have consented to be quoted in this book.

Various types of TN are represented, as well as different treatments that have been tried with different outcomes. Those quoted in this book offer their stories in the hope that they may reach fellow sufferers as well as speak to physicians serving patients with TN. *Trigeminal Neuralgia Exposed: "Our Story"* is a collaborative work, communicating the facts and fallacies that come along with the many facets of trigeminal neuralgia. May you read it in good health. And may it bring you hope.

Thanks to the Facial Pain Research Foundation and research scientists, for the first time in history research is being done to find the causes of trigeminal neuralgia, understand how it works and most importantly, find a cure!

All profits from the sale of this book will go to The Facial Pain Research Foundation for their continuing research. It is more than just for people with trigeminal neuralgia. These studies can and will impact many areas of neural pain care and may well be the greatest study and research into pain ever done. In studying the causes and nature of TN, a great deal will also be learned about nerve pain in general. The possibilities are astounding. **Just imagine!**

For more information, visit *FacingFacialPain.org*.

Contents

Disclaimers ii

Dedication iii

What is Trigeminal Neuralgia? 1

Facts and Fallacies 15

Other Facial Neuralgias and
      Possibly Related Conditions 31

Treatments 49

Trigeminal Neuralgia
      Surgeries and Procedures 61

Complementary, Alternative
      and Natural Treatments 73

How TN Changes Our Lives 85

Mental Health Care and TN 103

Hope 111

Organizations, Support
      Groups and Resources 119

What is Trigeminal Neuralgia?

What is Trigeminal Neuralgia?

The simple answer is that trigeminal neuralgia (TN) is a disorder of the fifth cranial nerve responsible for pain and other sensations of the face and is universally considered one of the most intense pains known to medical science. Beyond this simple definition, TN is a monster with many heads and tentacles.

The Studies

The Facial Pain Research Foundation was formed to find a cure and is already showing signs of being successful. Stem cell research currently underway has shown great success with the repair and treatment of neuropathic pain in the mice model. The Facial Pain Research Foundation is also conducting DNA studies to search for genetic markers that may predispose patients to trigeminal neuralgia. They like to call it "breaking the code to pain."

A third study at The Facial Pain Research Foundation seeks to figure out how the PMP22 gene normally works to help produce myelin and what happens in disease conditions to cause this gene to get stuck in nerve cells rather than traveling to the myelin sheath where it is needed. These, and more studies, are making our dreams of a cure come closer and closer to reality. The multi-pronged approach the Facial Pain Research Foundation is using is exactly what is needed.

The Trouble with Rareness

When a person is diagnosed with one or more rare medical disorders or orphan diseases, there are numerous problems that come into play. The following are just some of them.

Lack of Research and Funding: Research and funding for research in orphan conditions are one of the biggest battles rare conditions face. Most of the funding for rare conditions is generated by the fund raising efforts of patients and supporters.

Lack of Awareness (per June Toland Stephens): I worked in health care for many years, including as an emergency medical technician, and I had never heard of TN even though I was eventually diagnosed with it. I have met many nurses who have never encountered a patient with TN and/or have never heard of it. I have visited emergency rooms and have been seen by doctors who did not know what it was. Yet, beyond the medical world not knowing, it breaks my heart that many people out there may be suffering with this horrible condition and still not even know its name, much less what can be done for it. This, too, could happen to you.

Lack of Education: It would be impossible for every doctor to be taught about every rare medical condition. TN is no exception. We see a great need for our doctors to be better educated about TN. Much of the latest in research has not made it into the medical books. We would like to see continuing education offered on a wide scale to medical professionals in many fields.

Being Invisible: It is well known among patients with rare disorders or diseases that medical personnel are trained to look for the ordinary before the unusual. The adage is as follows: "If you hear hoof beats, think horses not zebras." This works for the many individuals that have common diseases and disorders, but it works against those who are afflicted with a rare disease or disorder, making them medically invisible, and their diagnosis can be delayed, ignored or missed. In fact, those with a rare disease or disorder can go misdiagnosed or undiagnosed for a number of years.

Our Medical Frustrations

There are many frustrations in dealing with trigeminal neuralgia. People newly diagnosed with TN are often overwhelmed with information that is conflicting, confusing and depressing. Some of the information they find can be misleading, outdated or incorrect. Or, they may find information that is merely the opinion of one neurosurgeon or neurologist on certain aspects of TN.

TN can be very confusing. It's fair to say most physicians have little education about trigeminal neuralgia. Many of us have encountered emergency room doctors that did not know what our condition was. And no wonder, they most likely only learned a paragraph or two in medical school. Surely it is frustrating to them as well. It's quite frustrating because neither the doctor nor the patient may know that they're dealing with TN. It's even more frustrating when a patient that has exhaustively studied the condition(s) is told things they know are outdated or inaccurate.

The Need for Up-To-Date Education for Doctors and Specialist

Very little is taught about trigeminal neuralgia and facial pain, and what is being taught is often based on old science that has been disproved or refined. While it might not be possible to educate all doctors about trigeminal neuralgia and other rare conditions, education on these conditions is an ongoing issue that must be addressed. The lack of knowledge and false understandings often combine to make it very difficult to get a proper diagnosis and treatment.

We would like to see more accurate education about trigeminal neuralgia offered to primary care practitioners. Continuing education on new findings and understandings of trigeminal neuralgia offered to all doctors, neurosurgeons, neurologist, pain management specialists and others will help ensure that health care givers are up to date on these important matters.

June Toland-Stephens: Yesterday, while in a store checkout line, I struck up a conversation with the shopper in front of me. During our short chat she revealed she was a nursing instructor. I had to ask, "Have you ever heard of trigeminal neuralgia?" She never had. Well, she has now. She said, "We can't teach it until they put it in the books." I asked her what she thought about continuing education being offer on TN and facial pain. She really liked the idea.

The Long Road to Diagnosis

June Toland-Stephens: In the front yard playing, an 8-year-old girl looks up at her older sister and asks, "Do you ever have pains in the side of your head?" The 10-year-old sister replies with a confused look, "Yeah, everyone has those." I know now that my sister was thinking about headaches. I remember thinking, "If everyone has them, I wonder why no one talks about them, cause that really hurts." At age 42, I was finally diagnosed with childhood onset trigeminal neuralgia, and I am by no means alone in this experience. Health care has come a long way since the 1970s, yet many people do go undiagnosed or are misdiagnosed today.

Alphonse Pellegrino: It took about six, maybe closer to seven years. I have Bell's palsy and synkinesis on the same side so my third through seventh cranial/facial nerves are shot. Still, no doctor would believe I had pain. One doctor that overheard me yelling at my regular doctor came into the exam room and said, "It's trigeminal neuralgia. Send him to a neuro consult."

Jenny LeCompte: Sigh. *Thirteen* long years of being misdiagnosed.

Lisa Malecha: I took two separate trips to the Mayo Clinic in Minnesota and never received a diagnosis. I had to go from Minnesota to Chicago to get a diagnosis. It took 10 years to get diagnosed. I was shuttled from doctor to doctor. I was angry for those 10 years, but when finally given a diagnosis, I felt scared yet relieved that finally someone figured it out.

Inadequate Medical Education and Its Toll on Our Medical Care

Our experiences range from comical, to sad, to life-and-death dangerous. One hope of this book is that it will find its way into the hands of many doctors, nurses and medical professionals, and that it will give them greater insights into the condition and those who suffer with it.

June Toland-Stephens: I think most doctors would agree that they don't get sufficient medical training about TN. Personally I have been in emergency rooms where the doctor did not know what trigeminal neuralgia was. Even among neurosurgeons and neurologists, we find that many have been taught information about TN that recent studies clearly dispute.

Gladys M. Rhodes: Going to the ER and the doctor whispering to me, "I know you are in a lot of pain, and I have no idea how to help. Do you know from past visits what has helped? If so, I can prescribe those meds and get you feeling better." This has happened to me four different times in Detroit! I really cherish these experiences.

Wendy: My doctor comparing trigeminal neuralgia pain to foot pain and wondering why Advil will not take care of the pain.

Christy Ritter: My last neuro said because I didn't have a tumor, I couldn't have trigeminal neuralgia. He said the pain was all in my head!

Alphonse Pellegrino: ER doctor ordered a chest x-ray for facial pain. I still have the report that says I'm complaining of facial pain and his order for the x-ray, and yes, I complained to the hospital about him.

Causes of Trigeminal Neuralgia

Mike Gaubert: Is trigeminal neuralgia a disease or a disorder? If it's a disease, then where did it come from and is there a cure? If it's a disorder, were you born with it? What body systems does it affect? Will there ever be a solution that successfully resolves the condition?

June Toland-Stephens: Actually, it can be considered both. There are many causes of TN, and often the cause is unknown.

Pat Zadorozny: Some of us got it after a facial injury.

Suzi Strand: I'm not 100 percent sure, but I have always suspected my TN and secondary progressive multiple sclerosis went hand-in-hand.

Kirsti Leeder: I never had mine confirmed, but my MRI showed that I had a buildup of fluid on the mastoid area of my skull from some sort of infection. The surgeon said it is possibly that, but he couldn't confirm it.

Kiley Burns: My MRI was clear, but then again, so was my mom's and she had a *bad* compression of the nerve. Both of ours started with dental work, so who knows. (Kiley and her mom both suffer from TN.)

Wendy: Trauma from a fall at age 43.

Kathy: My doctors don't know what caused my TN. It started eight months after major dental work including three root canals and five crowns. At the beginning of my illness in 2004, I went to the Scottsdale Mayo Clinic and had a $20,000 work-up—when I still had great insurance—to diagnose and rule out multiple sclerosis and many other diseases. All the test results came back normal.

Betsy Taylor Alexander: No clue what started mine.

Types of Trigeminal Neuralgia

A lot of confusion exists on the different types of TN. To this day, many neurosurgeons, neurologists and others who treat TN patients do not agree on the definitions of TN types. The definitions below were developed over time, are currently in use by many neurologists and neurosurgeons, and are being promoted for use to facilitate better communication between treating doctors and disciplines.

TN-1: facial pain of spontaneous onset with greater than 50 percent limited to the duration of an episode of pain (temporary pain). TN-1 causes intense electric-like strikes along the branches of the trigeminal nerve(s). Sometimes, TN-1 is also called classic TN or just TN.

TN-2: facial pain of spontaneous onset with greater than 50 percent as a constant pain. It is a constant burning type pain and may feel like crushing, ants crawling, knife searing or tearing pain.

Trigeminal Neuropathic Pain (TNP): facial pain resulting from unintentional injury to the trigeminal system, including facial trauma; oral surgery; ear, nose and throat surgery; root injury from posterior fossa or skull base surgery; and stroke.

Trigeminal Deafferentation Pain (TDP): facial pain in a region of trigeminal numbness resulting from intentional injury to the trigeminal system from neurectomy, gangliolysis, rhizotomy, nucleotomy, tractotomy or other denervating procedures.

Symptomatic Trigeminal Neuralgia (STN): trigeminal pain resulting from multiple sclerosis.

Postherpetic Neuralgia (PHN): pain resulting from herpes zoster (shingles) outbreak.

Atypical Facial Pain (AFP): If facial pain is not diagnosed by any of the categories above, it falls into the AFP category, which is pain that has no known physical cause and is thought to be psychogenic, generated by the brain itself, from a mental or emotional cause more than a physical cause.

Atypical Trigeminal Neuralgia (ATN): Many patients were diagnosed with ATN, an outdated term used before the above definitions were developed. Atypical meant that it was not TN-1 or typical TN. Most patients diagnosed with ATN have TN-2.

Source of the Types of Trigeminal Neuralgia: The Facial Pain Association and neurosurgeon Dr. Kim Burchiell of the Oregon Health & Science University

Anesthesia Dolorosa
Margaret L. Dennis, DMD

Anesthesia Dolorosa (AD) means pain (*delarose*) where there is numbness (*anesthesia*). It seems to be a consequence of too much damage to a nerve. It generally follows multiple procedures to treat nerve pain. It can happen in any nerve that is damaged. It is extremely odd as there usually is profound numbness, but still severe pain in the area. Trigeminal neuralgia is a disorder of the trigeminal nerve so yes, you can have both. You would have anesthesia dolorosa in the trigeminal nerve distribution. Anesthesia dolorosa usually trumps TN. There is no treatment available except pain management, because the nerve is too damaged by that point.

Melissa Waters: More so than the "real" pain, it's a haunting, aching, almost tingly pain that never goes away. It feels like there's an invisible vacuum drawing suction out of my lower teeth, molar area, and roof of mouth, which probably makes sense because I sustained chemical burns to my trigeminal nerve.

Christine Stefanik Spor: Yep, that's been my diagnosis for 14 years. Feels like a numb, burning, stabbing pain that is *always* there 24/7, 365 days a year!

Melissa Waters: I believe I've read about it. It has been referred to as Dantesque hell pain. It pushes you to your threshold of anxiety and sanity. God bless my good doctor for practicing compassionate medicine. And God bless my sweet band mates, Zipperneck Houston, for supporting me and distracting me from the hell every Thursday night. Surely there is a reason this happened to me. Just not clear yet what it is. I have devoted my life to taking pain away from others, both physical and psychological.

Kathy: I have anesthesia dolorosa resulting from gamma knife surgery back in 2004. I brought up this diagnosis with my neurologist a few years ago, and in his "humble opinion" he told me I don't have anesthesia dolorosa. How would he know if I have it or not?

What types of face pain are you diagnosed with?

Many times sufferers are diagnosed with TN without the diagnosis being specific as to type. From our support groups, we have found that TN sufferers often have multiple TN types or other facial neuralgia, as well as other neurological conditions, sometimes making diagnosis and correct treatment difficult and perplexing.

Barbara McDowell: atypical TN on the left side, occipital neuralgia developing, and TN may be developing on right side.

Wendy: TNP on the left side.

Alphonse Pellegrino: TN types 1 and 2 and occipital neuralgia all on right side.

June Toland-Stephens: TN-1, TN-2 and geniculate neuralgia on both sides.

The Types and Qualities of TN Pain

Many sufferers hurt constantly and only their degree of pain changes. Others experience pain randomly and in flares that can last hours, days, weeks and even months. Some have periods of remission or pain-free hours, days or even months. TN is also known to be progressive in nature. Remissions may come less often and/or disappear over time. From light stings to lighting strikes, burning like a sunburn to a raging fire, our descriptions are graphic.

Rebecca Thorpe: Imagine having your face and skull eaten by a huge bear—the crunching of the bone, tearing off muscle and ripping through the skin. That's my life with trigeminal neuralgia. Oh and the bear has a taser, too!

Christy Ritter: Constant pain, ice pick in my ear, stabbing knives that are connected to electricity, gremlins marching with spikes on my face. It's never ending. I could go on.

Pam Whitling Elliott: Constant prickly bee stings on the cheek with throbbing and burning in the sinus area. Stabbing in the eye socket is a chronic electric shock that is also a chronic headache. All of this goes on the pain scale at never less than a two all the way up to a 10. I also get quick jolts of electric shocks in my teeth, tongue and lip. Once in a great while, I feel like bugs are in my nostril.

Allison Ramirez: I have bilateral atypical trigeminal neuralgia on all six branches, and the pain never stops. It varies in intensity, but some part of my face is always painful.

Wendy: Constant burning pain under my eye, cheekbone, upper lip and side of nose, as well as in my nasal cavity. When it flares, it gets worse in those places, but also starts hurting in the teeth (upper, sometimes lower), deep in the eye and also on the lower lip. The constant pain is burning and aching. As it gets worse, the aching leaves, and it is pure burn with some stabbing quality. Once amped up, the pain stays high for a number of hours or more, regardless of what I do or don't do.

Mike Gaubert: In my jaw I get rapid successions of lightning bolts (short term) or extreme pain lasting 12-plus hours. In my zygomatic arch, I get extreme pressure and pain lasting four-plus hours. In my left temporal area, I feel lightning bolts and a sharp, ice-cold steel spike being shoved in there every few minutes. My left nasal cavity and nose has sharp, shocking pain when touching it and when breathing through it. My mouth and gum line have sharp pains when breathing in cold air. All of the above may last up to 12 hours without relief. The left side all at once—crushing, sharp pain with lightning bolts lasting for up to 14-plus hours. Then there are the one-sided headaches not relieved by anything except a Dilaudid injection in the ER or Percocet 7.5/325 mgs and three Aleve by mouth, if taken early enough.

Kiley Burns: My pain is 24/7, 365 days a year with lightning bolts in my teeth, jaw, cheeks, TM joint and occasional shocks from my temple to my eye or in my ear. I only have the shocking type pain, but it never goes away. I don't have "attacks." The pain is always there in the same way, but the intensity can vary. My mom is the same way.

Barbara McDowell: My pain is 24/7, and it's been like this for about a year and a half. Well, I did have a few days here and there that were pain free. Most days are not bad, about a five or lower. Sometimes they are higher, and once in a while they are off the charts.

Kathy: I have pain 24/7, 365 days a year, going on 11 years now without one second of pain relief since it began on March 5, 2004.

Patti: Mine usually takes turns. One day it's my right eye, down my nose and into my upper lip. The next day, it's all in my left cheek. I also have bilateral occipital neuralgia that never stops. The doctor basically says the muscles in my neck and shoulders are paralyzed and one nerve sets off another nerve, it tells two friends and so on and so on.

What are your triggers?

Some people find that heat triggers or increases their pain, while others are able to use heat to ease their pain. It is these and other paradoxical factors that often make TN a very difficult condition to treat because what helps one person may hurt another.

Anything can trigger an attack or make the pain worse. We spend our days trying to avoid the many triggers of TN. A cool breeze has the power to bring us to our knees. We fear kissing our mates, children and grandchildren because it can bring on excruciating pain. Some wrap their faces in scarves against the wind, cold and heat. Some have such hypersensitive pain sensors that even wrapping soft scarves around their faces is too much. These pain triggers often leave us feeling isolated from the world, and the list of activities that must be given up is staggering and life changing.

Betsy Taylor Alexander: Wind, stress, cold on my face, brushing my hair, washing my hair, loud noises like music that's too loud, touching my face, washing my face. . . . Should I continue? LOL!

Debbie Murphy: Stress, wind, change of weather, particularly if the pressure is going one way and the temperature is going another (and I live in the Midwest), kissing, touching my face, brushing my hair, taking a shower, my nose running, the fabric touching my face when I wrap it, brushing my teeth, eating, even on the other side, and so on.

Allison Ramirez: Life. It's constant and everything affects it—the weather, barometric changes, wind, solar events, grooming, eating, exercising, talking, singing, sneezing.

Jenny LeCompte: Wind, cold, direct sunlight, change of body temperature in any extreme, stress (ugh stress), brushing teeth, dental work (the *thought* of dental work, LOL!), my hair getting out of a rubber band and touching my face—even the slightest bit, chewing, high pitched sounds, stress. Did I mention stress? We should all be given a lifelong refillable prescription for Ativan or something like it as soon as we get diagnosed!

LeeAnn Ryan: Everything, just everything.

Facts and Fallacies

Facts and Fallacies

Fallacy: Trigeminal neuralgia usually strikes individuals over 50.

June Toland-Stephens: When I first started studying everything I could find on trigeminal neuralgia in 1998, the thought was that trigeminal neuralgia primarily strikes people over age 70. Then in a few years, it went to age 60. Now, most available information says over 50. The truth is there are no accurate statistics, so we do not know. Because TN has different causes and is progressive, it stands to reason that it will appear more among the older population, rather than the younger. Still, this causes many children, youth and young adults with TN to go undiagnosed or to be misdiagnosed.

Gladys M Rhodes: I was diagnosed at 29. When I had my microvascular decompression surgery at age 36, my surgeon informed me that the damage to the nerve was so extensive it probably started when I was 8 years old!

Jenny LeCompte: First pain was at 15 years old. I was not diagnosed until I was 27. It started on my left side, but has since progressed to bilateral.

Kaleigh Roberts: I was diagnosed at 27 years old, earlier this year.

Alphonse Pellegrino: Well, I will kill two myths; I'm under 50 years old and I'm male. I was diagnosed about two years ago at age 48, but I've had trigeminal neuralgia, types 1 and 2, since 2007.

October 7, 2015 is our Third Annual International Trigeminal Neuralgia Awareness Day. This year, it is dedicated to our youth and children that have TN.

Children get trigeminal neuralgia too!
by Chris Nolze

Hi, my name is Chris Nolze, and I was first diagnosed with trigeminal neuralgia two years ago at age 16. Finally getting a doctor to correctly diagnose me took a long time, though. We endlessly went to every doctor that we knew at several of the top medical centers in New Jersey, New York, Philadelphia; you name it and we went to these medical centers in the hopes that somebody would figure out my trigeminal neuralgia. Each stop seemed like even more of a letdown. Time after time, every doctor either said that I was faking the excruciating pain for attention or that my parents and I made the whole situation up to get pain medication.

We did find one neurologist in Philadelphia that said my case seemed to be pediatric trigeminal neuralgia, but he said that there was nothing he could do. Due to my age category as a pediatric patient at the time of my onset of TN, I was caught in a situation that shouldn't exist. The pediatric neurologists were not properly trained to deal with trigeminal neuralgia in pediatrics, and the adult neurologists wouldn't see me because I wasn't old enough. The sad fact is that since going through my situation, I have seen more and more fall into this category where neither doctor will touch the case.

We finally ended up finding a doctor at John's Hopkins, in Maryland, and he was the first doctor that could actually help. Under his care, I underwent a rhizotomy, along with two microvascular decompressions (MVDs)—one on each side. However, after my second MVD, I had post-op complications and ended up requiring reconstructive surgery due to an infection on my skull. I ended up with a large titanium plate replacing a portion of the right side of my skull, and I wasn't really the same afterward.

One night at dinner a few months after my reconstructive surgery, I randomly got the hiccups. At first, it seemed normal and just mostly annoying, but as the night went on I realized they weren't going away. I went to bed and the next morning when I woke up, they were still there. Over time they got faster in frequency and got to the point where I was hiccuping about 200 times per minute. By a freak of nature, a friend of ours found that a TENS (transcutaneous electrical nerve stimulation) unit stopped the hiccups only when placed at the exact spot where my titanium plate was in my head.

For over a year, we traveled across the country looking for a doctor to help, which was a lot like our experience with trigeminal neuralgia. Again, all of the doctors told my parents and me that I was faking it for attention or pain medications. We went to the top-notch hospitals, from John's Hopkins and the Cleveland Clinic, to the Mayo Clinic and multiple hospitals in New York. Nobody listened and meanwhile I was literally living with the TENS unit taped to the side of my head. Without it, the hiccups were so frequent that I could not breathe.

As an absolute last resort and last option, a friend gave us the information for a doctor in California. We sent a video of the hiccups to him and he said that he wasn't completely sure what was taking place, but he was willing to see me. So at the last minute, we booked a flight and flew out to California, unsure of what he would say or find. We saw Dr. L. on a Monday and right away he ordered a special type of MRI that would show if there were any compressions on my cranial nerves; it is the same MRI used sometimes to diagnose trigeminal neuralgia. We had been pleading for doctors to do this for about a year, but they all said that it wasn't necessary and that I was faking my symptoms to get out of college—mind you, I still maintained a full course load.

That same week on Wednesday, I had the MRI and by Friday Dr. L. had a game plan. The MRI showed that I had two major arteries pushing on my brain stem along with uncountable amounts of compressions on my other cranial nerves. Around the same time, my trigeminal neuralgia had also returned full force and the MRI showed compressions that were left on my trigeminal nerve as well.

Dr. L. went ahead and did an MVD on each side. On the right side, he went from cranial nerve #5 up to cranial nerve #10, along with my brain-stem, moving and cushioning endless amounts of compressions on my nerves. About two weeks after the first surgery, Dr. L. went in on the left side in order to decompress my trigeminal nerve, but the surgery actually took just as long as the one on my right side, due to the extreme amount of scar tissue built up.

My case with trigeminal neuralgia and with the hiccups is very rare. I am only the third reported case of intractable hiccups in medical publications, and I will be the first to have any sort of follow-up care. My trigeminal neuralgia was very rare because it was constant, bilateral and returned. The largest and most important part, I think though, was the struggle that we had to go through to find a doctor to listen. Dr. L. was my last hope and thankfully he was willing to listen and help. He found out that the only reason the TENS unit was working the way it did was because the titanium plate was thinner than my skull, so the electric signals were able to reach my brain, similarly to how a deep brain stimulator works.

If it weren't for Dr. L. and the TENS unit, I'm not sure what kind of shape I would be in today or if I would even be alive. This experience has taught me two things: Doctors need to be made more aware of these issues, such as pediatric trigeminal neuralgia and intractable hiccups, so that others can be treated, and doctors need to listen more to their patients. I saw far too many doctors that instantaneously wrote me off as a psychological case and said it was stress. There needs to be more proficient care and treatment, and doctors should not write off patients, as so many TN patients have experienced.

Things I wish someone would have told me when my daughter was diagnosed with TN

by Stacie Winslow

1. Trigeminal neuralgia is progressive and will get worse. Pain will get more intense, periods of remission less frequent, and outbreaks will last longer, *despite* increasingly higher doses of medication.
2. Just because a compression isn't visible on an MRI doesn't mean there isn't one there.
3. All neurosurgeons are not equal. They all *learn* to perform MVDs, but that doesn't mean they *should* perform them. Doctors have to stay current and be experienced in the procedure.
4. Some of the ear and eye pain associated with trigeminal neuralgia *could* be caused by compressions on other cranial nerves.
5. Most surgical treatments, other than the MVD for trigeminal neuralgia, are palliative. They treat the symptoms, but the pain will likely reoccur.
6. Nerves *can* remyelinate themselves once compressions are removed.
7. The amount of medication she is taking will sneak up on you. As you fight to control the pain and add more and more medication, you will lose parts of your child.
8. Progression of this disease is not a failure on your part. As time marches on, it will get harder to deal with the pain. When medications stop working, it isn't your fault.
9. Try anything. Try everything. But be very cautious of expensive treatments that promise too-good-to-be-true results. I feel many of us (yes, us!) start throwing money at solutions or give up hope once we are told there are no visible nerve compressions.
10. Never stop searching. An answer, a cure, hope is out there.
11. Dentists are good people and we all need them, but trigeminal neuralgia is *not* a dental problem.

acy: Trigeminal neuralgia pain is always caused by nerve compression(s).

Many were told it wasn't trigeminal neuralgia because no compression(s) of the nerve was seen on a regular MRI. The importance of checking for compression(s) must be seriously emphasized. It is highly recommended that anyone with trigeminal neuralgia get a FIESTA MRI or a trigeminal neuralgia protocol MRI in order to better visualize the compression(s), should there be any. An MRI is also needed to rule out multiple sclerosis and other possible factors that might be causing trigeminal neuralgia.

It is still generally believed that trigeminal neuralgia is mainly caused by one or more compressions of the trigeminal nerve, however new studies are raising questions. Dr. Burchiel at Oregon Health & Science University has discovered that approximately 17 percent of the mature population has one or more compressions of the trigeminal nerve, while less than one percent of that group ever develops trigeminal neuralgia. This is a clear indication that some other mechanism is at work. Currently, studies sponsored by the Facial Pain Research Foundation are underway to help uncover what these mechanisms may be.

Research scientists believe that their DNA studies may explain what predisposes a person to this condition and what makes the nerve misfire. Just imagine how many people this study could impact. One of the most amazing DNA studies in neural pain is being undertaken at the Oregon Health & Science University, in Portland, OR, by one of the principal researchers in the Facial Pain Research Foundation's trigeminal neuralgia project. One hundred participants with trigeminal neuralgia type 1 (TN1) have been enrolled and their DNA gene samples have been collected. There are an additional eight DNA collection centers located throughout the United States, Canada and England. Obtaining the DNA samples and supporting the collection centers is extremely important to the project.

Fallacy: Opiates never work on trigeminal neuralgia.

Many neurosurgeons, neurologists and pain specialists were taught that opiates don't work on trigeminal neuralgia or nerve pain, but new studies show that opiates work for some patients with these conditions. One such study can be found at: ncbi.nlm.nih.gov/pmc/articles/PMC4133425.

It must be stressed that every person is different, and what works for one person may not necessarily work for the next, but then again, it may. Every person responds to medication differently, opioid or not. We want our doctors to remember this and give sufferers an opportunity to try the opiate medication and see if it will work for them. Because the pain can be so intense, a person may need stronger dosages of opiates, or any other medication, to be effective. For some individuals with addiction problems, opiates may not be the best choice.

While many find opiates to be very helpful, others are helped more by anti-seizure medications. The most recent studies are recommending the use of both. However, the side effects of both anti-seizure medications and opiates may limit a patient's choice to one or the other.

Nothing written here is to be construed as in any way condoning drug addiction, but being medically dependent on pain medication and being an addict are two different things. Today, it seems that both types of patients are treated with the same kind of disrespect. Opiates are not the answer for all people with TN, and of course there are inherent concerns with all opiate use. However, in light of the current swing away from opiate use, it is important to acknowledge opiates as one of many treatments that should be considered for trigeminal neuralgia.

Alphonse Pellegrino: I take Oxycodone and Tramadol, when needed. They take away some of the constant pain, plus I'm on Carbamazepine twice a day, every day.

Dianna Vanderburg Demay: Yes, opiates help. I take Opana. I have TNP.

Suzi Strand: I found opium helpful. Opiates helped to take the edge off breakthrough pain. However, being a chronic pain patient, they don't prescribe them to me. Percocet worked decently enough.

Jennifer Click: Dilaudid is my savior. No side effects. No sedation. In fact, if I take it too late in the day I will toss and turn all night. Only medicine that helps, but I won't get it again after this script runs out.

Gladys M. Rhodes: Doctors tried all kinds of medications, and they didn't work. Opiates came to my rescue for 11 years.

Important points about opiate use with trigeminal neuralgia.

There are dangerous and life threatening side effects from opiates, but that's true for non-opiate TN medications, as well. Addiction can happen to pain sufferers, and self-control or even external controls are important. However, it has been shown that addiction among true pain sufferers is not common. Like many others with pain conditions, people with TN experience the effects of the war on drugs and often feel like the prisoners of war of that battle.

There are different types of opiates for different needs, including immediate release, extended release and abortive or rapid onset opiates for emergency or extreme attacks. If the dosage of opiates is too low, it will not work, and this could fool many into believing they do not work at all. Many times a second pain medication is needed for breakthrough pain.

Dear emergency room doctors and staff:

I come to the ER complaining that I'm having pain on the side of my head.

My face is unwashed. (It hurts us to wash our faces.)

My hair is uncombed. (It hurts to comb our hair.)

My teeth look an awful mess. (It hurts to brush them, too.)

I rate my pain a 12 on the 1-to-10 pain scale.

I'm very anxious and my jaw twitches here and there (facial tic).

Am I a drug addict? I realize I look the part, but the answer is no. I have trigeminal neuralgia.

Fallacy: Trigeminal neuralgia is usually unilateral; pain is only felt on one side at a time.

June Toland-Stephens: I'm going through the bedroom door when two lightning bolts strike on the right side, branches two and three. Then, one on the right side strikes. Now all three branches on the left have TN-1 and TN-2, both going nuts.

Allison Ramirez: I'm so sorry, I agree. Both sides are bothering me today. Don't you want to just smack anyone who says that it isn't bilateral and that both sides don't fire at the same time?

Debbie Murphy: I've actually just had that happen (bilateral) a few times and thought I was losing my mind, but it's seriously only been a few times. This year was the first time it was bad enough for me to admit I was bilateral.

Anne Plohr Rayhil: Well, it's interesting and timely you ask, as I have bilateral pain. My right side bothers me much more than the left. It is extremely rare for both sides to hit me at the same time. Doctors will tell you this doesn't happen at all, I'm sure. However, yesterday I "ate" lunch with friends. They of course picked a seat outside on a beautiful sunny day. The breeze was slight, so I wore a protective scarf. I ate the soup. Then I started to get twinges, then burning on both sides. I got into my car and the heat from my car and a breeze hit me full force. Holy crap! Burning, zapping, V1, V2 left side and all three branches on the right side. The Emperor from Star Wars was apparently hiding in my car, and I didn't know it! Once I pulled myself together, I called my mother to come retrieve me, and I waited in the cool of the restaurant until she arrived. The rest of the day was more of the same. I am a bit better today, but I'm terrified of setting things off. Ugh, what a way to live.

Rebecca Webb: It takes me to my knees when both sides hit together.

Amy Popovich: My left is the main side. When it hits both sides, the pain can be so severe that I am barely able to interpret it. I just close my eyes and the pain seems to bounce around between ears, nose, cheek, teeth and eyes. The eyes are the worst. Even with my eyes closed, I can see flashes of light in various forms that seem to pound with each heartbeat, swish swish swish—a terrifying sound echoing in my ears because I know what comes next

Fallacy: Trigeminal neuralgia can't kill.

June Toland-Stephens: TN has threatened my life at least three times.

First incident: I had a bad flare going on, and by the third morning the strikes were hitting at their worst and I kept getting chest pains. I called 911 and while I was in the ambulance and hooked up to a heart monitor, a lightning-bolt-strength strike of pain went through my face. Immediately, I felt chest pain and the alarm went off on the heart monitor. The medic repeatedly asked me, "Do you have a pacemaker; do you have a pacemaker?" I answered, "No, it's the TN strikes in my face." He said, "It looks like your heart is being shocked by a pacemaker." I have never had any heart problems before. This raises a serious question about the risk to someone with a heart condition who also has TN. Interestingly, the ER brought me out of this crisis with 2 mg of Dilaudid and 2mg of Ativan. In my opinion, this refutes the thought that opiates do not work on TN-1. That day, they may have saved my life!

Second incident: In addition to TN, I have three cerebral aneurysms. I've laid in the ER watching my heart rate on the monitor make huge spikes, in perfect timing with the strikes in my face. The harder the strike, the higher the spikes went. The next morning, I called my neurosurgeon that was overseeing my aneurysms and spoke to his nurse. I told her what had happened and asked her how dangerous it was for my aneurysms. Her answer: "Very! That's worse than if your heart rate went high and stayed there."

Third incident: I was feeling fine with no pain and had just sat down at the computer when I was suddenly hit with a monstrous pain strike. I blacked out, only for a few seconds, and then came back to full consciousness. But then I was hit with another strike and blacked out again. This happened three times in rapid succession. I yelled for my daughter to call 911, but by the time I got to the hospital and was examined by a doctor, the beast had gone back into hiding.

It stands to reason that the intense pain suffered by people with TN can raise blood pressure. This and the other stresses that the TN pain puts on a person's system can seriously affect many underlying conditions. Short or long term side effects from the medications can also be fatal. People with TN have passed away due to over-medication as well as suicide. Trigeminal neuralgia may not kill directly, but trigeminal neuralgia *does kill*!

Trigeminal Neuralgia Progression

People that have progressive trigeminal neuralgia will experience longer bouts of pain and shorter periods of remission. When previously only one area of the face was affected, now other areas of the face will have pain. Or, there may simply be increased pain, tingling, burning, stabbing and other symptoms in all of the affected areas.

Jenny LeCompte: One of the most challenging parts surrounding this incredibly difficult illness is that after 20 years, (heck after just a couple years, even when I was a young child) I would tell my doctors that the pain, year after year, was getting worse. There is no data to back this up, yet I've heard many other people say the same thing. When I see my doctors, they are not always in agreement. I try to make sure the doctors know that I have done my research and that I'm not just blowing smoke because I am the one who is living with this illness!

Sarah Edmondson: I know that my pain has progressed since the beginning; even the bad episodes are different. I do think mine has progressed into my occipital nerve, at least according to my doctors

Suzanne Martin: I can add here that my TN has progressed the last three years. I have had trigeminal neuralgia for 13 years and it has never really been under control. I am lucky in the sense that my neurologist acknowledges TN progression. He informed me! He was so right.

Wendy: My trigeminal neuralgia progression has been subtle yet real. From the distinct trigeminal neuropathic pain pattern on the V2 branch, now involving the V1 branch, and sometimes the V3 branch, all on the left side, going on for over 14 1/2 years. Doctors at the 2013 San Diego International Trigeminal Neuralgia Facial Pain Conference acknowledged the progressive nature of this as being basically common knowledge, however my neurologist looks at me cross-eyed when I mention this progression. I keep educating him; fortunately he appreciates the education.

Debbie Murphy: This past fall after five years, I was suddenly struck with what must have been trigeminal neuralgia progression. It was like one day I was so much worse, and I haven't gotten better. During these past few months, I visited the emergency room for the first time since my initial diagnosis.

Kimberly Marin: Mine started in my lower branch on the right side. It worked up to the middle branch and finally to the upper branch (V1). Now I've been having pains on the left side. I also developed occipital neuralgia after gamma knife surgery. I'm in remission now thanks to gamma knife surgery, but I have been feeling pin-prick pains on my left side for the last two months.

Kiley Burns: Mine started in my lower left and right branches (V3) and then moved to the middle branches (V2) on both sides. It next moved to the top branch (V1), right side, followed by the left side. This progression happened in a year's time.

Christy Ritter: Mine started with pain on the right side in my cheek bone, and it has now spread to all three branches—bilateral in one year!

Allison Ramirez: I have atypical trigeminal neuralgia (ATN). It started over 20 years ago with pain in the second branch (V2) every winter. We thought I just had sinus issues. Then the V3 and the V1 branch over my left eye went off with a continuous headache, and it didn't stop for more than ten years! Now it is in all three branches, bilateral. The pain varies in intensity, presentation and on which branch or branches it flares, but the pain never stops.

Barbara McDowell: Mine is mostly on the left side, upper two branches (V2 and V1). Sometimes, the lower branch (V3) joins the hellish party. Every once in a while, I experience zaps in all three branches on my right side. They thankfully are very few and far between. The doctor has said that I am now developing occipital neuralgia.

Betsy Taylor Alexander: Mine has finally gone to all the branches on my left side. It started along my jaw and teeth (V3) and moved on to my eye. Every now and then, I feel something weird on the right side and it scares me that it is moving over there, as well.

Debbie Murphy: Mine started in all three branches and has continued that way for almost five years. It has now been affecting the top two branches of the other side.

Alphonse Pellegrino: Every once in a while, my jaw on the other side will start to twitch and feel like it's being cut. I would not be surprised if I get it full blown on both sides; it's just my luck. Bring it on trigeminal neuralgia. I will fight even harder to survive. I will not fall!

Pam Whitling Elliott: Mine spread because of the multiple procedures I tried to stop the initial pain. It woke up the other nerve branches. Ouch! Mine stayed in the V2 branch on the left side for years until I had glycerol injections, and then it seemed to damage or weaken the V3 branch on the same side; I had pain from that for several years. I then had a radio frequency procedure done, and that affected the V1 branch, which caused constant strikes and chronic headaches. Between the injections and radio frequency procedure, I also had a microvascular decompression (MVD) which failed. I then went on to have the nerve partially severed, but it still didn't stop the V1 pain strikes. My progression didn't spread on its own. It was caused by injuries due to surgeries and procedures.

Other Facial Neuralgias and Possibly Related Conditions

Other Facial Neuralgias and Possibly Related Conditions

More often than not, trigeminal neuralgia appears to come with company. Very few of us suffer from TN alone. Some of the different types of facial neuralgias and possibly related conditions are: glossopharyngeal neuralgia, occipital neuralgia, geniculate neuralgia, Bell's palsy, cluster headaches, migraines, temporomandibular joint disorder, and many others. A few of these are highlighted in the following section.

Geniculate Neuralgia

Geniculate neuralgia (GN) arises when the nervus intermedius, a small nerve, is compressed by a blood vessel, resulting in severe, deep-ear pain, which is usually sharp—often described as an ice pick in the ear—but may also be dull and burning. This ear pain, which may be accompanied by facial pain, can be triggered by stimulation of the ear canal, or can follow swallowing or talking. For more information, visit: *upmc.com*.

June Toland-Stephens: It's funny how our friendship and support for each other evolved. I must thank Lisa Malecha, who made this important point: With all the attention that TN is finally getting, it is important to also include other facial pain conditions. She told me about geniculate neuralgia, indicating that I should look it up, which I did. I then realized that the many hours I spent in emergency rooms believing I might have an earache that was aggravating my TN, was probably geniculate neuralgia. I now understand that along with childhood TN, the earaches I had as a child were geniculate neuralgia. I promised her that in spreading awareness, I would include other facial pain conditions.

Lisa Malecha on Geniculate Neuralgia: The definition of geniculate neuralgia is that the artery is compressing the seventh cranial nerve instead of the fifth cranial nerve, like in TN. Four days after I gave birth to my daughter, I developed Bell's palsy. I had all the symptoms of

Bell's palsy plus severe ear pain and pain down my jaw. I couldn't even listen to my daughter cry because it aggravated the pain. Actually, I couldn't listen to my daughter for her first five years because she had what we called a Minnie Mouse type of voice.

After seven months, the Bell's palsy went away and I was left with this pain in my ear and down my jaw. It felt like someone shoved a pencil in my ear and was trying to move it around. Other times, it felt like an ice pick poking inside my ear. It was almost constant and so severe that I wanted to just take a knife and slice off my ear and dig up my eardrum. I would get so dizzy and couldn't walk straight. After the Bell's palsy went away, I was sent to the Mayo Clinic in 2002, and the first neurologist I saw said it sounded like the seventh cranial nerve. The doctors at the Mayo Clinic said it was atypical facial pain and possibly TN-2, and I was put on a medicinal regimen. That was the last mention of the seventh nerve for a long while.

As I continued to bounce from doctor to doctor, neurologist to neurologist, and finally surgeon to surgeon, I was just beyond frustrated. Eight years had now passed, and I had made a second trip down to the Mayo Clinic. Now they wanted to put in a brain stimulator. The surgery sounded so scary, and I just couldn't see myself going through it. I had been seeing a pain doctor for about a year, and he suggested I see a new surgeon, so I reluctantly went. Well, lo and behold, he didn't feel there was anything to be done. My current MRI showed nothing. He saw my disappointment and suggested I go down to the University of Illinois, in Chicago, and see a surgeon who specialized in surgery on cranial nerves. Sure, why not? What did I have to lose?

I had never been to Chicago, so we made a mini-vacation out of it with the kids. They had a blast, but I had one thing on my mind. My appointment was a nightmare. I waited an extra hour in the waiting room and almost two and a half hours in the exam room. I was ready to leave. Finally he came in and examined my MRI, shook his head and told me he just didn't see anything. I started to cry. This was sort of my last hope. He then stopped and said, "Wait a minute. I'll be right back!" He came back 15 minutes later, looked at me and said, "You have geniculate neuralgia, a compression on your seventh nerve, and we can fix that." Well, you can imagine the relief. I felt like I lost 100 pounds off my shoulders. I finally had my MVD three months later and he actually decompressed my 7th and 8th nerves. He found my 8th nerve also was compressed when he was fixing my 7th, even though it never showed up on my MRI.

Unfortunately, I was only pain-free for three months. I also am now deaf in my left ear because they went too far down the nerve. They said they could have gone farther, but were afraid they would make me deaf, so who knows, maybe another MVD will help. I also had to have ear surgery to help with balance and dizziness. However, the pain in my ear is much better, just not the rest of the left side of my face. I still get ear pain, just not as often. So back to the beginning, every neurologist I had seen in those ten years labeled me as atypical facial pain; now we know I had geniculate neuralgia for the past 16 years and will have it for the foreseeable future.

As many can proclaim, once I had the final diagnosis, I felt like a huge weight was lifted off of me and I didn't feel like I was crazy. I used to be on 27 medications on a daily basis to help with the pain, but I'm slowly working my way off some. Geniculate neuralgia is pretty tricky, and it always seems to poke through several times a day, along with some TN-2. My story just keeps going on from year to year, and every year it's a little different as it progresses.

Occipital Neuralgia

Occipital neuralgia (ON) is a distinct type of headache characterized by piercing, throbbing, or electric-shock-like chronic pain in the upper neck, back of the head, and behind the ears, usually on one side of the head. Typically, the pain of occipital neuralgia begins in the neck and then spreads upwards. Some individuals will also experience pain in the scalp, forehead, and behind the eyes. Their scalp may also be tender to the touch, and their eyes especially sensitive to light. The location of pain is related to the areas supplied by the greater and lesser occipital nerves, which run from the area where the spinal column meets the neck, up to the scalp at the back of the head. For more information, visit ninds.nih.gov/disorders/occipitalneuralgia/occipitalneuralgia.htm.

Kimberly Marin: My trigeminal neuralgia came first; I got occipital neuralgia from my gamma knife surgery. Recently, my TN pain has been coming back, and I have had stabbing on the top of my head, aching in the back of my head and shooting pains down my neck, followed by shocks in my teeth and stabbing pains in my cheek or eye. At the moment, my head feels like it's in a vise, pressure all the way from the top of my eyebrow over the top of my head, down the backside and down my neck with needle prick stabs. I often get migraines from occipital neuralgia because sometimes it is so constant, and as mentioned above, it sets off my TN. It hurts to lay my head down; I put muscle rub behind my ear, down my neck and on my forehead, just for some slight relief.

Christy Ritter: Mine pretty much came together, I think. I fell, hit my head and had a seizure. Finally in January 2012, after years and years, I was diagnosed with occipital neuralgia, and in April 2012, trigeminal neuralgia. It took forever just to be diagnosed! Most of the time for me, both are flaring at the same time. I get blurry vision a lot, just like today with my right eye, I couldn't see anything and my left eye is blurry; plus it feels like needles in my eyes. At times the occipital neuralgia burns and it feels like I'm being scalped, but I also get electric shocks. With TN my whole face burns and I feel electric shocks, ice pick in my ears, needles in my eyes and throat and giant hot searing needles in my cheeks.

Wendy Gray Meek: My ON attacks come with no warning. My vision is affected during an attack; I get blurry or no vision in my right eye. I have bilateral trigeminal neuralgia, but my right side is my worst.

Anne Plohr Rayhill: I got occipital neuralgia from having microvascular decompression surgery for my TN. The surgery incision was gigantic and cut across or close to the occipital nerves on the lower right side of my head. I have tons of scar tissue in the occipital region.

Multiple Sclerosis

Approximately five percent of patients with TN have multiple sclerosis (MS), and about two percent of patients with MS will develop TN. Approximately 85 percent of patients that have both MS and TN will develop additional MS symptoms before the TN, and an MS diagnosis is usually established before they develop TN.

Patients with MS are about 20 times more likely to develop TN than patients without it. Patients with TN and MS are more likely to be younger than those without MS. Patients with TN and MS are more likely to develop TN on both sides of the face (approximately 20 percent of patients) than those without MS (approximately 5 percent of patients), but it is rare for anyone to have it on both sides of the face at the same time. For more information, visit *trigeminalneuralgia-ronaldbrismanmd.com*.

Jennifer Click: Multiple sclerosis is a very interesting disease, especially if you don't have it. The average age of diagnosis is 33. If you lived your first 15 years above the longitudinal line that runs through Tennessee and around the world, you are more likely to develop this disease. Multiple sclerosis is not found in third world countries. It also tends to be a middle-class disease. The reason it's termed "multiple" is because there are multiple symptoms that go along with it. Where demyelination is found on the myelin sheath that covers the spinal cord or nerves in the brain determines what symptoms you may have. Scarring and lesions are just another term for demyelination. Those of us with multiple sclerosis who also have trigeminal neuralgia may have demyelination and scarring on the trigeminal nerve. Or, we could have trigeminal neuralgia completely apart from multiple sclerosis.

Suzi Strand: Just like with trigeminal neuralgia, there are different versions of multiple sclerosis. My TN isn't caused by compression(s) and I have no lesions on my trigeminal nerves. They think the trigeminal neuralgia is from myelin degradation, just like my multiple sclerosis.

Temporomandibular Joint Disorders

Found on either side of the head in front of the ears, the temporomandibular joints are two pairs of joints that connect the lower jaw to the skull and allow the jawbone to rotate and slide. These joints allow us to talk, chew and yawn. When one or more of them becomes inflamed or painful, the condition is called temporomandibular joint disorder (TMJD or TMD). For more information, visit *cedars-sinai.edu/Patients/Health-Conditions/Temporomandibular-Joint-Disorder-TMJD.aspx.*

Margaret L. Dennis, DMD: Saying I have TMJ is like saying I have a knee because it just names a joint, rather than a condition of the joint. TMJ is an out-of-date term; we can be *much* more specific nowadays. A more appropriate and collective term for any facial pain that might be connected to the temporomandibular joint is TMJD.

The TMJ is a ball-and-socket joint, just like other joints in your body. There is a cartilage disc between the bone of your skull and the bone of your lower jaw. If that disc is damaged or displaced, it can cause pain and limited growth of the lower part of the jaw. You use your jaw to speak, swallow and chew, so doing any of those activities can be painful.

The only connection between TMJD and trigeminal neuralgia is that the TMJ is innervated by the trigeminal nerve. Damage inside the joint can mimic trigeminal neuralgia pain. It is easily distinguished, though, using an MRI of the temporomandibular joints to show the damage. Additionally, a block of the temporomandibular joint can be performed, and if the joint block decreases the pain, then surgically correcting the damage may reduce the pain.

If the case is truly just trigeminal neuralgia, no damage to the temporomandibular joint will be seen on the scan. This is important because if the facial pain is treated with typical treatments for trigeminal neuralgia, such as gamma knife or MVD, the actual source of the pain (the TMJ disorders) will not be treated and the pain will continue. I am afraid this is the reason for failures of some MVDs. Anyone with facial pain and/or headaches should have their temporomandibular joints imaged. There is no other way to diagnose a temporomandibular joint problem!

Manuela Bradshaw: Thanks for the TMJD information Dr. Dennis.

Dennis L Wiant: I was never diagnosed with TMJ disorder, with no dental insurance, but I know I have it. It is very annoying and painful on both sides. On the right side—my TN side—sometimes it's hard for me to tell the difference if it's TMJD or trigeminal neuralgia with ear and jaw pain.

Betsy Taylor Alexander: I had TMJ disorder really bad in my early 20s, but I wore an appliance in my mouth that changed my bite and actually pulled my lower jaw out a bit. I don't have any more popping, dislocation or the debilitating headaches!

Christine Stefanik Spor: I was diagnosed with TMJ disorder as well; it's what started my trigeminal neuralgia problems!

Margaret L. Dennis, DMD: A damaged temporomandibular joint can cause facial pain like trigeminal neuralgia, but if the pain is coming from the joints themselves, it can be fixed by repairing the damaged joints. TMJ problems can only be diagnosed by MRI, remember that. It just makes good sense to rule out TMJD before proceeding with other measures.

Rebecca Thorpe: I have severe popping on both sides and have crushed my four back molars into powder from clenching my jaw as I'm being shocked by TN, although nothing shows up on the MRI that can be corrected. I'm supposed to get a splint to help keep my face relaxed during an attack, but my insurance doesn't cover TMJ splints, which can run into several thousand dollars. Seems TN makes TMJD worse and TMJD makes TN worse; so I'm just kind of stuck between a rock and an electric fence.

Dennis Gannon: I've had severe TMJ all my life, and around 2005 it really started to hurt.

Bell's Palsy

Bell's palsy is a form of facial paralysis resulting from a dysfunction of the facial cranial nerve VII, causing an inability to control facial muscles on the affected side. Often, the eye in the affected side cannot be closed. The eye must be protected from drying up or the cornea may be permanently damaged, resulting in impaired vision. In some cases, denture wearers experience some discomfort. The common presentation of this condition is a rapid onset of partial or complete paralysis that often occurs overnight. In rare cases—less than one percent—it can occur on both sides, resulting in total facial paralysis. For more details, visit *en.wikipedia.org/wiki/Bell%27s_palsy*.

Bell's Palsy and Trigeminal Neuralgia
Q and A with Jenny LeCompte

How old were you when you had your first Bell's palsy symptoms?

It was November 3, 1993. I had just turned 15 a few months prior.

What type of trigeminal neuralgia do you have?

Looking back, I know that my TN started on my left side only as TN Type 1 and progressed into TN Types 1 and 2 within the first few years. About 15 years later, it has become bilateral with TN Type 1 and 2 developing on my right side as well.

What were your first symptoms of Bell's palsy?

On November 3 1993, I got up and went to school like any other day. I was a sophomore in a very small high school in Pleasant Hill, Oregon. I remember sitting in my first period class and noticing that my left eyebrow felt, well, funny. It would have a bit of a twitch or a muscle spasm of sorts. I remember thinking how weird it was that my eye would start watering, and if anyone was looking at me from the side they would easily think I was crying out of my left eye only. For some reason, tears started running down my cheek, but I had no control over it whatsoever.

So, as I sat there working on my math test and anxiously awaiting the bell to ring, I could feel my face getting that blushing feeling because I was sure everyone was noticing that my eye was looking and feeling so strange. Once the bell rang, it was on to my second period class. As the day went on, so did the strange feeling in my face. It was like someone drew a line straight down the middle of my face; the left half was completely affected. As I sat in my second class of the day, my nose started bothering me. I had a sensation like my nose was running even though it was actually fine. I felt as if I needed to wipe it every few seconds.

So I went on with my day. By my third class, I remember I was sitting next to my best friend and we were whispering back and forth, even though we were supposed to be listening to the announcements for the day. I was trying to ask her if anything looked strange with my face and was telling her about what had happened during the first two classes. As soon as I said something about how it felt and we both started laughing, she suddenly stopped, looked at me and said, "Jenny, *stop*! That's *not* funny." As soon as I asked, "what?" I could feel that my face, including the left side of my mouth, had now "dropped."

For some odd reason, I didn't even ask to leave class. We just sat through class, and as soon as the bell rang, I remember my best friend looking for a few of our other friends to see if they would come look at my face. No one had seen anything like it—we were only 14 to 15 years old, after all. Looking back, I wish I had asked to see the school nurse, or even to go home for the day and asked my mom to get me into the doctor quickly or just, in general, had more concern over what happened. But because I didn't feel any major pain in the very beginning—if anything my face felt numb in the beginning—I had no concerns.

Where on your face did it start and/or spread to?

It definitely happened over a period of several hours and *definitely* was affected much like the branches of the trigeminal nerve are separated. Starting with the top branch then progressing down until all three branches were affected and paralyzed. Because my case was considered quite severe, I still have residual effects in the top branch; I can only move my left eyebrow if I *really* concentrate on trying to move it, and it has been that way ever since I was 15. When I have recurrences of Bell's palsy, the strangest part to me is that it can be all three branches or it can be just the top branch or just the bottom (third) branch.

How did Bell's palsy progress? How did trigeminal neuralgia progress? How are they interwoven?

My Bell's palsy progressed over the course of that first day, and for approximately one year thereafter, I was unable to move the left half of my face. I couldn't blink or close my left eye; I was constantly checking my mouth because I felt like I was drooling; I had to learn how to eat again without food falling out of my mouth; I had to learn how to drink again out of the right side of my mouth—to this day, I can only drink with a straw.

I was told very early on that "typical" Bell's palsy episodes last anywhere from three days to three months and that if it lasted longer than that it was most likely permanent. After about a year, I was able to begin moving my face again. It started with twitching around my lower eyelid and the corner of my mouth, and took a lot longer to get to the point where I could move my face as much as I'm able to today, but it happened and it did make me wonder why the doctor was so sure I wouldn't be able to move it again.

I remember my mom taking me back to the doctor, and when we asked why it was that I could now move my face and why there was *so* much pain involved as well, his answer was one that I still ponder to this day. It's honestly the reason I believe there are such things as miracles and unexplainable experiences—medical or otherwise. He told us that after a nerve becomes paralyzed for a period of time—apparently over three months—it will basically "die off and shrivel up." He went on to explain that there was the potential that if even one cell of the nerve was still "alive" that it could end up "regenerating" and branching back out into my face and causing a type of nerve pain known as neuropathy.

Neuropathy was the diagnosis I was given for 13 years until I got the *real* answer as to why I was in so much pain. I learned about neuropathy and knew it was a general description of nerve pain, and I also knew in my gut that this was not just neuropathy.

The TN progression is harder to describe in depth, as I wasn't even diagnosed with TN until I was 28 years old. That said, I do remember the pain bringing me to my knees from the very beginning when I was 15. As time went on, doctors had me keep pain journals every time I felt like I was being hit by lightning or stabbed with an ice pick over and over again. I would mark the time down and make a "mark" based on the intensity of the pain.

Over time, the pain has definitely progressed from only TN 1 on my left side to both TN 1 and 2 on my left side for the first 15 years. Now, after years, it has become bilateral. My left side is definitely worse, as that side has been affected longer than the right side, and I'm not sure the right side will ever "catch up" to the same degree of pain, intensity or frequency.

Looking back, the hard part is that I personally used the pain as a driving force in my life. I worked two to three jobs at all times up until I had my son. I went to school and graduated with five degrees, including a bachelor's degree in psychology and a master's degree in educational leadership. I bought my first home by the age of 22 and was raising my son on my own at age of 25. Because I had endured many tests and had so many specialists tell me I was crazy, or that something must have been going on at home and that I was seeking attention, I got to the point that I knew I needed to keep the pain inside of me and not show that it bothered me as much as I could. I am *not* saying this is a good way to cope. In fact, I do not suggest it at all, but it's how I managed, and if I had to do it over again, I would most likely do it the same way.

What were your first trigeminal neuralgia symptoms?

The first symptom I had was the feeling of being stabbed in my ear, deep, deep in my ear canal with an ice pick, over and over again. This was the night before my face was paralyzed. I remember thinking, "I've never had an ear infection before and cannot imagine that they are *this* painful." Now looking back, I know that very first pain was actually the first trigeminal neuralgia pain that I had. With Bell's palsy, all the symptoms took place within the first several hours and now that I have recurrences, they are very sporadic and typically when I am very, very stressed, have gone without sleep for a long period of time or just for any reason that my fifth or seventh cranial nerve decides to go off. It definitely has a mind of its own, much like trigeminal neuralgia.

During an attack, how do the two play off each other?

It's hard for me to always be able to differentiate which one is affecting which. Honestly, because they both originally took place at the very same time, it's a lot like the old question, "Which came first, the chicken or the egg?" I will say that having the recurrences of Bell's palsy and becoming a pro at figuring out what my triggers are for my TN, there are a few things I am more than certain of. Stress, lack of sleep and any major change in my typical routine, or even of the weather, absolutely affects both my Bell's palsy and my TN. If I were to track how I had been feeling with regard to my TN before a Bell's palsy attack, more than likely you'd see a correlation: The worse the pain is, the more likely the Bell's palsy is to act up and/or last longer.

Due to Bell's palsy complicating your condition, how long did it take to get diagnosed with trigeminal neuralgia?

It took 13 years from the time the trigeminal neuralgia began until I was actually diagnosed with TN. Since the Bell's palsy and trigeminal neuralgia started at the same time, and honestly I believe that because Bell's palsy is something people can *see* visually, it was taken more seriously than any pain I was in. Doctor after doctor insisted that Bell's palsy does *not* cause pain. That is fine, but there was still the fact that I was in *so* much pain. My mom and I were told, visit after visit by doctor after doctor, that I was not in pain and that I was making it up. It is *so* complicated and the *only* thing that makes me feel any amount of validation is the fact that I did finally get a diagnosis.

I had just about given up on ever having a *real* diagnosis or reason for my pain after 13 years of seeing neurologists and being treated for "facial neuropathy" that was believed to be a result of the severe case of Bell's palsy.

Ultimately I was at the end of my chances of being treated with medication when one day I was reading the local newspaper, I'm not sure if all papers have a *Dr. Doctor* section, but it's much like *Dear Abby*, only medical. The subject this day was about facial pain, and the words "trigeminal neuralgia" were right there in black and white. The person who wrote in was concerned about their adult child's facial pain and the medications they were using to help it. The medications were *all* the same medications I had tried. For some reason, I just *knew* this was my answer. Even crazier is that as I began to tear the article out, my phone rang with my mom calling to tell me that I needed to read the *Dr. Doctor* section of the paper. I told her I had to go; I had just read it and needed to call and make an appointment with my neurologist.

I had been seeing a neurologist for migraines, and he would discuss my facial pain, but ultimately I had begun feeling like it was a lost cause. When I went in to my appointment the CNA who was taking my vitals asked if it was a migraine I was coming in for, and I anxiously took the article out of my pocket and showed it to her telling her I wanted to discuss this with him. I will *never* forget her almost audible gasp as she told me, "You do *not* want that disease!"

And I'm thinking, "Um, no, I don't *want* it, but I believe I have it." She went on to try and tell me I needed to do some research about it before I talked to him about it because, "it's called the Suicide Disease and we have a patient in the hospital right now because she's unable to speak or chew food; it's horrible." Those words would stick with me forever. After all I had been through with doctors she worried me enough that I almost didn't talk to the doctor about it, but I decided I was there and that if nothing else I wanted it ruled out. There had to be something they could do to test for it.

Well, as I talked to my doctor about it he tried to tell me there was "no way" I had trigeminal neuralgia. I was too young, he said. At this point, I was 27 and *still* considered too young. I was never someone who would stand up to a doctor or any medical professional, but something in me told me to advocate for myself like never before. I told him I wanted whatever test I needed, if I didn't have it, fine, but I wanted it ruled out and I wasn't leaving until he agreed. He wrote the order for the MRI and explained that I would never have had this specific MRI before, even though I had already at this point had *many* brain MRIs over the last decade, because it is in a specific area they have to look at.

I went to my MRI and got a call the same day saying I needed to come in to discuss the results. There is something interesting about being a "professional patient" and I'm sure it helped that I had worked in medical settings, but I knew that if the results are 'fine' or nothing major they just tell you that over the phone. If it's bad news, they make you come in for the results. Strangely, this didn't concern me all that much. I went in, and as I waited for the doctor to enter the room I wondered if this would be the chance I would finally get to fix this pain. As he entered the room, he chuckled seeing it was me and said, "Well, you were right. I was wrong. It is trigeminal neuralgia." He explained that I had already been on all the medications for neuropathy, which would be the same medications that would be tried for TN, and he suggested that I go see a neurosurgeon to see if they could perform a brain surgery that could fix my pain. I felt excited.

Validation. I was *not* crazy. The pain was *real,* and there was a reason for it. My artery is wrapped around my trigeminal nerve, compressing it in several places as the artery was wrapped around the nerve multiple times. My neurologist even went on to tell me how the radiologist who looked at my MRI actually called him and had him pulled out from seeing another patient, because he was "so excited" about my MRI. I had to ask him to clarify "excited." Apparently TN is rare. Rare enough that it's not something every radiologist will even see in their career. It was all so surreal.

That day changed my life forever. I wanted nothing more than to have a copy of that MRI to take to every specialist I had seen the previous 13 years. I didn't go this route, but I do still consider it, not out of anger or spite, but out of concern for others out there who are not being listened to because they are too young or any other reason. I've heard it all. I still hear it all the time. "You're too young to have issues like this." Ummm, that doesn't change that I *do*. It feels insulting, as if I had anything to do with making myself "alter-abled".

There is no other reason for my TN. There wasn't trauma—it wasn't from having surgery, dental work or any other reason that some people end up with TN. Now that I have a diagnosis, I ask any doctor I see what they know about my TN and why I got it as well as Bell's palsy. On *multiple* occasions and by multiple doctors I have been told it's just "bad luck." And the fact is, it doesn't matter *why* I have it, I want a cure. I need a cure.

We All Deserve a Cure

Lisa Malecha: My TN and Bell's palsy came at the same time. The doctor was puzzled because there shouldn't be pain with Bell's palsy. When it went away, after seven months, the pain stayed.

Jennifer Click: It seems like many of those with TN may at some point get Bell's palsy. I had two episodes, and the medical staff thought I was having a stroke. I was treated with a steroid for 10 days and each time I got better.

Kim Stephens: I didn't have TN and Bell's palsy together. I had Bell's palsy about a year before TN. But I believe that some things that happened after the Bell's palsy was really my TN starting, although not yet full blown, if that makes sense. I've always felt that the Bell's palsy is what caused it, and now after being told they think the nerve is damaged, I'm even surer. You don't really read much about Bell's palsy causing TN, but I have read it and was told by a doctor it could be the reason. For months, I suffered with burning ear and pain mostly around my cheek and in my eye. I just thought it was a relapse and that the pain in the face was just from the pulling on my face from the paralysis. I now have bilateral TN-1 and TN-2. It started on my right side, and within the last two years it has gone to my left side; my left side doesn't have the constant pain as much as the right side.

Treatments

Treatments

Treatments for TN can often be just as grueling as TN itself, be it the anticonvulsants, opiate pain medications, injections to the nerves or one of several different types of procedures or brain surgeries. They all carry risks.

Medications

Many types of medications are used to treat TN, and it is important to understand that often multiple medications will be needed to manage TN pain. As of this date, no medicine has been designed specifically for TN...*yet*! As of October 2014, there is a new TN drug being designed that is in third-phase trials and has been given orphan drug status.

"An orphan drug is a pharmaceutical agent that has been developed specifically to treat a rare medical condition, the condition itself being referred to as an orphan disease. The assignment of orphan status to a disease and to any drugs developed to treat it is a matter of public policy in many countries and has resulted in medical breakthroughs that may not have otherwise been achieved due to the economics of drug research and development." Wikipedia contributors, "Orphan drug," *Wikipedia, The Free Encyclopedia*, wikipedia.org/wiki/orphan_drug (accessed October 20, 2015).

Common Trigeminal Neuralgia Medications

Anticonvulsant Medications

 Tegretol: generic name is Carbamazepine

 Carbatrol: generic name is Carbamazepine; extended release

 Trileptal: generic name is Oxcarbazepine

 Topamax: generic name is Topiramate

 Phenytoin: generic names are Dilantin and Phenytek

There are many other anticonvulsant medications that a doctor may choose to try.

Neuron Stabilizing Medications

    Neurontin: generic name is Gabapentin

    Lyrica: generic name is Pregabalin

    Savella: *Warning*! This medication may cause high blood pressure problems.

Opiate Medications

Many other opiates are available; these are only the most widely prescribed.

    Oxycontin

    Methadone

    Percocet

    Morphine

    Hydrocodone

    Fentanyl patches

    Fentanyl Buccal tablets: They dissolve under the tongue.

Some neurosurgeons, neurologists and pain specialists were taught that opiates do not work on TN or nerve pain. Newer studies show that opiates do work for some TN patients. For more on this, visit *ncbi.nlm.nih.gov/pmc/articles/PMC4133425*, as well as *ncbi.nlm.nih.gov/pmc/articles/PMC3411376*.

Other Medication

    Baclofen: muscle relaxer

    Klonopin: generic name is Clonazepam; commonly used for anxiety. It is also helpful with some types of nerve pain.

    Ativan: an anxiety medication also used for neural pain

Many people with TN also suffer from anxiety, post-traumatic stress disorder and depression due to their TN. Many also have mental health issues not directly related to TN but which TN can cause to escalate.

As with other pain conditions, treating the mental health issues of pain sufferers is very important to pain management. Many people have found the following medications as well as others to be helpful.

Anxiety Medications
Klonopin

Ativan

Xanax

Valium

Anti-Depressant Medications
Lexapro

Cymbalta

Celexa

Depakote

Many medications have been tried with success for some and failure for others. Often it is a case of weighing the side effects against the benefits. Sometimes the medications work at first but become less-effective or ineffective at all over a period of time. A medication may work for one person while showing no benefit whatsoever for another sufferer.

Our Best Medication Combinations

The following medication combinations are what we and our doctors have found to work for us. The information contained here is not intended to replace your doctor's advice. Please be sure to follow your doctor's recommendation when it comes to medications and medical advice. *Always be safe*! Always read the medication inserts and never be afraid to ask questions about your medications.

Suzanne Martin: Oxcarbazepine, Topamax and Citalopram. High dose of the first two and low dose of the third one.

Wendy: Oxycontin, Topamax, Cymbalta and Klonopin. I use non-time release Oxycodone for flares, all at low doses; each one works on different brain centers. I would love to learn more about cannabis for TN. *[NOTE: since the original notation, Wendy no longer uses Klonopin. The CDC studies uncovered distressing data implicating Klonopin, possibly in combination with an opiate, in a disturbing number of deaths over a short length of time.]*

Rebecca Webb: Tegretol, Amitriptyline, Valium, Lortab Norvasc, Stadol nasal spray, Promethazine, Antivert, Zoloft, Ambien and Flexril. I also use a motor cortex stimulator for pain control. That's enough for three people.

Suzi Strand: Cannabis and Kratom

Christy Ritter: I have been on Dilantin, Depakote, Topamax, Trileptal, Lexapro, Effexor, Gabapentin, Tegretol, Amitriptyline and Lyrica. I haven't found a combo that works for me.

Medication Side Effects and Dangers

Allergic reactions can happen to anyone! Side effects can be very mild or non-existent in one person and in another be life threatening or fatal. Many of the TN medications we are prescribed are very harsh, as our sufferers can attest to. In addition to the short term side effects, we also need to consider the long term effects, which are not pleasing at all. Always read your prescription inserts. If you don't understand something, ask your doctor or pharmacist to explain it. Mixing medications as we sometimes must do can be a very dangerous game.

Side Effects

Rebecca Webb: Tiredness, dizziness, the jerking is a mess and my eye crossing. I can't stand any of these.

Alison Ramirez: Fatigue, lethargy, slow thinking, loss of memory, weight gain, edema, dizziness and loss of emotional control.

Rebecca Thorpe: It would be easier to say what the medicines don't do. With the three that I've been on, side effects are: vision and hearing impairment, unsteady gait, kidney damage, speech difficulty, balance problems, night sweats and weight gain. I can't drive; I'm always cold but sensitive to heat; and I have memory loss, which is why I can't remember the other side effects.

June Toland-Stephens: With Neurontin I had a functional black out. I woke up on a bus with the driver telling us to get our IDs out because we are crossing the border into Canada. I didn't remember leaving work on Mercer Island, WA. With Tegretol, my stomach automatically rejects it, and Lyrica gave me panic attacks.

Kiley Burns: Tegretol made me sick to my stomach, dizzy and exhausted. I wanted to sleep all the time when I wasn't busy throwing up. I switched to Neurontin, and now my only side effects from any of my medications are some memory loss from the Neurontin and constipation from the pain medications. I had no side effects even while adjusting to the Neurontin or raising the dose; I'm lucky. They had to do the same for my mom's Fentanyl. She was on 150 mcgs every other day, changing them earlier than normal and a higher dose than normal. The doctor had to fax a signed waiver.

So Many Bottles
by Allison Ramirez
12/6/13

So many bottles
So many pills
Take this they say
To cure your ills

They come with friends
That change your brain
Scramble your thoughts
Make you feel insane
What should help
Just makes you sicker
Slows your mind
Your thoughts get thicker

There is no cure
I have no choices
These pills I take
To still the voices

Of pain and despair
Loneliness and fear
Grief and sadness
The skull head leers

Laughing mocking
Only to prove
These pills make it
So hard to move

It's all a lie
The promise they make
Every time they give me
Another pill to take

Trapped I am
In this vice of pain
I give up too much
To feel well again

Procedures

With procedures, as with the surgeries and medications, some sufferers find help from them while others find little or no help at all, and in some cases the procedures can cause further harm.

Injections or Nerve Blocks

Neurolytic agents provide a longer time of pain relief, typically lasting for a few months. They achieve this by causing destruction of nerve fibers, degeneration of axonal fibers, and Schwann cells. The neurons regenerate in three to five months. Often, it might take one to two weeks before complete pain relief is experienced. For more information, visit emedicine.medscape.com/article/2040595-technique.

The neurolytic agents used in trigeminal nerve blocks include the following:

Glycerol: This agent is typically used for treating TN. It is a mild, neurolytic agent, but it can also cause perineural damage.

Alcohol: Currently, this agent is rarely used, because of its high rate of complications; it can seep into surrounding tissues and cause necrosis and cellular injury, and it can also cause vasospasm.

Phenol: This agent is also commonly used. It can cause warmth and numbness on the injection site, and it can cause convulsions and cardiovascular collapse if inadvertently injected intravascular.

Botox, steroids and other numbing medications are also sometimes used as injections to treat TN.

Neuro Stimulation

From stimulator wires placed in the spinal column and wires placed directly on the face, to the P-Stim in which wires are connected to points on the ear lobes, there are many types of neuro-stimulation being used with TN, including motor cortex stimulation; which we will discuss under brain surgeries.

There are many different stimulation treatment options available. The P-Stim stimulation treatment option is highlighted below, particularly due to its noninvasive method. Sheri Neumoyer began trying the P-Stim during the Summer of 2014. Thank you, Sheri for sharing this experience with us.

P-Stim

Sheri Neumoyer, with the help from Matt Williams, Sheri's caregiver, shares with us some information about her P-Stim for trigeminal neuralgia.

I have atypical facial pain and TN-2 on the left side. But the P-Stim may help patients with Type 1 or 2. The stimulator is self-contained with the battery and is glued behind the ear then covered with tape. They used a wand that finds the strongest nerve activity closest to the skin. There are three small needles, one in my ear lobe, one near the opening of my ear and the other in my face right next to my ear. It's incredibly noninvasive.

I had a little mishap with the first one, so technically I had it installed on Tuesday, May 27th, 2014. It's worn for four days and then off for three days. You actually remove it yourself and throw it away. The doctor installs a new one each week. After four weeks, it's supposed to have lasting effects and you no longer wear it.

I had this done at Merritt Island, Florida. I had been going to the same pain center in Philadelphia, PA since December 2004 and was terrified of finding a new doctor. I may have gotten lucky and found a good one on the first try!

Unfortunately, Sheri's insurance stopped paying for her P-Stim. She reports that with the P-Stim, she did have a lower level of pain and was able to function better. It helped her stay out of bed more.

P-Stim Questions Answered by Sheri Neumoyer's Doctor

Has the P-Stim been successful in lowering pain levels for both TN-1 and TN-2 patients?

Yes

Are you collecting statistics on trigeminal neuralgia patients using the P-Stim?

Yes. I'm in the first year of collecting stats on the P-Stim. I would like all my trigeminal neuralgia patients to try it because it's so simple and there's effectively no risk.

How would you treat a bilateral trigeminal neuralgia patient?

Bilateral patients wear the P-Stim on one side the first week, then switch it to the other side the next week.

Trigeminal Neuralgia Surgeries and Procedures

Trigeminal Neuralgia Surgeries and Procedures

Any surgery is a scary thought. Brain surgery can be even more terrifying. Among our different Facebook groups, in any given week, there may be several people facing brain surgery. For some people, it could be their first, second, third or even fifth brain surgery.

Others may be facing the heart-wrenching and very difficult decision-making process of whether or not to have surgery, or they may be debating which brain surgery is best for them. Brain surgery works hard on the mind.

Radio Frequency Thermal Lesioning

Radio frequency lesioning, also called radio frequency rhizotomy, can be a good option for high-risk patients, such as patients with concurrent illnesses that would make an open surgical procedure too dangerous. It can also be a good option for patients with multiple sclerosis whose TN is often not caused by vascular compression. Radio frequency lesioning does not treat the root cause of TN but instead selectively destroys nerve fibers associated with pain and damages the trigeminal nerve to stop the transmission of pain signals. If necessary, the procedure can be repeated.

Balloon Compression

Balloon compression may successfully control pain in some people, at least for a period of time. Most people undergoing this procedure experience some facial numbness, and some experience temporary or permanent weakness of the muscles used to chew. This procedure is performed under general anesthesia.

Micro Vascular Decompressions

Compression of the trigeminal nerve is the most well known cause of TN. When a compression is found it is most often a vascular compression of the trigeminal nerve, close to where it exits the brain stem, but compressions can occur anywhere along the nerve and often other cranial nerves are also compressed.

Compressions can sometimes be hard to see and are often missed by regular MRIs. It is suggested that people with trigeminal neuralgia or facial pain should have the new, high resolution MRIs, sometimes called a FIESTA MRI, 3D thin slice cut MRI, TMJ MRI, or trigeminal neuralgia protocol MRI, which will show a compression much clearer. Your neurosurgeon is the best person to order your MRI as he knows the correct one to order.

Micro Vascular Decompression (MVD) is the only surgical option that doesn't intentionally damage the nerve. MVDs are done under general anesthesia. During the operation, an opening is made in the skull just behind the ear. If a blood vessel is found pressing on the trigeminal nerve, a soft piece of Teflon is placed between the vessel and the nerve, lifting the vessel away from the nerve.

MVDs are most effective on TN Type 1. While in cases of compression(s) this may be the best option yet, the fact remains that decompression can only help if that is the cause of the neuralgia. Some TN sufferers have had an MVD attempted, but no compression(s) were found.

MVD Comments

Anne Plohr Rayhill: My TN was caused first by an arterial compression. Actually, an artery was splitting my nerve apart, but that wasn't visible until surgery. Pain relief was noticeable and blissful right after surgery. However, the surgeon placed a Teflon pad that was too big so my results were short-lived. I started having some shocks four months later. It took me almost two years, two neurologists and two neurosurgeons before I was taken seriously. I had a second MVD in Peoria, Illinois, where scar tissue was found compressing my fifth, seventh, and eighth cranial nerves. I now have hearing loss as a result.

June Toland-Stephens: My MVD helped, but it didn't stop the pain by any means. The painful storms that used to last up to eight days now last at the longest, three or four days. Other than that, everything else is the same. I am grateful for that. The surgeon didn't find any clear compressions, yet he did place a Teflon pillow on a suspected artery and he cut out a vein that wasn't supposed to be there. I have bilateral TN, but I have only had procedures and surgeries on my right side.

Betsy Taylor Alexander: I was told that my TN is caused by a compression of a vessel on a nerve. During the first MVD the surgeon placed the Teflon pad between the vessel and the nerve. During the second MVD the surgeon didn't find a compression, but he did something else in there. He didn't explain it to us, so I need to get my surgery report. He told me that the vessels are always curling and moving around as we age and that it's likely I'll have another compression. Well, I guess that time has come.

Cathy McKinnon: I have trigeminal neuralgia, atypical trigeminal neuralgia, plus nerve damage from MVD surgery. My MRIs were clear, but my doctor was willing to try anyway. Our family was praying so hard for him to find something that could be fixed instead of him saying he didn't see anything wrong. In 2008 when I had my MVD, I was having around 100 to 150 jolts a day. When I woke up from my MVD they said an artery was found pressing on the nerve, so he put the Teflon padding between the artery and the nerve and also clipped a blood vessel that was floating at the nerve. When I woke up, the jolts were gone. One of my ministers was standing there when I woke up and he said, "You are smiling. I've never seen you smile before." It was absolutely wonderful to not have the jolts.

After some time in recovery, they put me in a large private room with around-the-clock nurses for my personal care. My doctor preferred it that way instead of the ICU because he believed that it was best not to be around all the ICU noises and that personal care in a private room was best for recovery and healing. I was there four days. I had no complications and did exactly as instructed for the six weeks of recovery. When I went back to the surgeon he said he knew I still suffered from the atypical trigeminal neuralgia and nerve damage, but I looked like a different person. He also commented that I was smiling, and he never saw me smile before. Yes, my MVD was successful and I wish you and everyone else could be as blessed as me.

Kiley Burns: My mom's MVD was 15 years ago, and it failed. Her MRI was clear, yet when the surgeon did the surgery, she had a large artery compressing the nerve so badly and for so long, that there was permanent damage to the nerve root. They put a spacer in anyway, but the pain didn't get any better after the surgery. She also had a severe cerebrospinal fluid leak in the hospital and was bedridden for two months before she was able to even go downstairs to the kitchen. It was a very rough recovery and while it failed, she doesn't regret doing it. She never would have known whether it worked or not without at least trying. She was 35 years old at the time of the surgery and had already had TN for approximately 10 years.

Lisa Malecha: My MVD was a complete disaster. Not only did I wake up from surgery deaf in one ear, but a month later I had to go back into the hospital for another surgery to fix the first one. The first surgeon used a surgical glue to put my skull back together and it began to leak. Not only did I end up with a staph infection, spinal meningitis and the worst headache ever, but a different surgery pulled some fat from my stomach to seal the skull permanently. The wound in my stomach, as well as the meningitis and staph infection kept me in the hospital for 31 days. My white blood counts were never in the normal range, so they struggled fixing that. I had two spinal taps and more blood work than you can imagine (always at 4:30 in the morning...lol), but finally after 31 days I was able to go home with a home-care nurse. So now I had a failed MVD and needed a nurse to come every other day to check the wound in my stomach. One time she made us go back to the ER because I was running a high fever, but that didn't last more than a day. So I have experienced more pain then I ever imagined since my MVD.

Kirsti Leeder: I had my first MVD on the right side in 2009, but it didn't make much difference with the pain. I had my second MVD in 2012, and I was in the hospital for five days (compared to five weeks for the first MVD). I was off all medications before I left the hospital. I guess I spent the first couple of weeks constantly thinking it was going to return, but it didn't. I felt I could be "normal." I could do all those things that everyone else takes for granted—going out in the breeze, playing with the children in the snow. The only thing that bothered me was a pseudomeningocele over the wound.

After about 18 months, I noticed little signs that it was returning. To be honest, I ignored it for three months as I did not want it to be true. On the fourth month, I had to admit it was back and had to re-start medications. I was completely gutted. I now have hydrocephalus as well.

Christine Stehanik Spor: I had my MVD in 2003, and it did not work for me. Unfortunately, I woke up with a damaged nerve.

Stereotactic Radiosurgery/ Gamma Knife Surgery

Gamma knife radiosurgery (GKS) is a minimally-invasive treatment that uses targeted beams of radiation to treat tumors and other abnormalities in the brain. GKS does not involve surgical incisions, so it's generally less risky in many ways than traditional neurosurgery. For trigeminal neuralgia treatment, the radiation beams are aimed at the trigeminal nerve near where it enters the brain stem and focuses close to 200 tiny beams of radiation at the nerve. Gamma knife treatment does not target the root cause of trigeminal neuralgia, but instead causes mild damage to the trigeminal nerve to stop or reduce the transmission of pain signals. Although each beam has very little effect on the brain tissue it passes through, a strong dose of radiation is delivered to the site where all the beams converge on the trigeminal ganglion close to the brain stem.

Early complications or side effects are usually temporary and may include fatigue, swelling, and scalp and hair problems. Months after GKS, some people may experience late side effects, such as other brain or neurological problems. GKS is especially appropriate for older people who have other health problems and cannot have open-skull brain surgery.

GKS is usually an outpatient or overnight procedure, and recovery time is usually minimal. You will have a team of three doctors: a neurosurgeon, a doctor of radiology and a nuclear physicist. Before the procedure begins, a special frame will be attached to your head with four screws. You will receive numbing shots in the four places on your scalp where the pins will be inserted.

Two pins will be on your forehead and two at the back of your head. This frame will stabilize your head inside the gamma machine during the radiation treatment and serve as a point of reference for the beams of radiation. You may ask to be given pain medication if the placement of the frame causes your TN to flare.

After the frame is attached, you will then undergo an MRI of your brain that shows the location of the nerve in relation to the frame. The MRI scan will then be used to select the target area for treating your TN. Because the treatment is so precise, there is little exposure to surrounding healthy tissue.

The results of the brain scans are fed into a computerized planning system that enables the surgical team to plan the dosage of radiation to be used and the appropriate areas to treat, and to map how to focus the radiation beams so that they treat the nerve without causing harm to other vessels. This planning process may take an hour or two. During that time, you can relax in another room, but the frame must stay on.

During the procedure you will lie on a bed that slides into the gamma knife machine, and the head frame will be attached securely to a helmet inside the machine. The procedure will take about one hour.

You'll be able to talk with the doctors via a microphone. You can listen to music. You won't feel the radiation.

After the procedure, the head frame will be removed. You may have minor bleeding or tenderness at the pin sites. You will be able to eat and drink after the procedure. GKS creates a lesion to block transmission of pain signals along the trigeminal nerve. Pain relief may take six weeks to several months to be effective.

Gamma Knife Surgery Comments

Jane Harris Kelley: I've had six and a half years of pain relief from gamma knife surgery, and I am 15 months medication free.

Kathy: I had gamma knife surgery in 2004, and it did not help me. In fact, it damaged my left eye. Now I have pain in my left eye, and it hurts to open it. I also have chronic dry eye.

June Toland-Stephens: My gamma knife surgery helped to reduce my pain considerably for about nine months.

Motor Cortex Stimulator

My name is Rebecca Webb and this is my story. I have TN, atypical TN, occipital neuralgia (ON), and glossopharyngeal neuralgia. I was born this way. I believe the ON is from the migraines I have suffered with for 14 years. It took six neurologists 10 years to diagnose the problems and the next four years to try and correct them. I've had two MVDs done by the same neurosurgeon. They relieved some, but not all, of the pain. I have two vented plates and eight screws.

I went to another neurosurgeon, and he offered me the option of the gamma knife surgery. I would have had to wait for six months to see if it worked. If it didn't work, I would have had to stay in major pain for the rest of the six-month period. So, I went with the motor cortex stimulator.

So off I went to get this done. The first part of the motor cortex stimulator surgery process was a mapping MRI to see where they would place the electrodes. The second step was to open my skull to place the electrodes and wires on the opposite side of the trigeminal neuralgia. They placed the electrodes on the dura mater layer of the brain and threaded the wires through a hole placed in the bone.

When in recovery I noticed that the wires were hanging out. They cut my head from the top to just below my ear with staples all the way down. I went to neurosurgery ICU until the next day. The doctors came in to check on me, and they tried the stimulation, and it worked. *It worked!*

All I could do was cry; not being able to say anything, the doctor knew it was working. He had tears in his eyes, which made me cry more. He told me if I ate lunch I could go home, and to be back the next week to place the rest of the wires and the battery. I couldn't eat lunch, but did get some food in later that day. I was soon home.

Next, all I did was rest, and my friends came to make sure that the staples looked intact. The next week they opened my head and put more wires in from my neck to my chest where the battery was to be under my skin. It sure felt like liposuction and was very sore as well. Back I went to neurosurgery ICU where I stayed until the next day.

The Doctors came back with a bag full of equipment I would be using. There were several pieces, which was confusing for me at first: one item to charge the battery and another to charge the charger. The next day i was moved to another room. I went to sleep that night and woke up with a swelled face. The nurse called the doctor to come look at me. I had to stay sitting up to see if it would help; no changes. The bruising was from my head to my breast. The doctor said if I ate I could go home after dinner. I was so glad to go home. I had learned a lot on my own with the stimulator.

The bruising was gone after several months. Three months later, I needed adjustments, so off to the doctor's office I went, and again several other times after that. It has helped with the ice picking stabs and shocking pain. But I still have days when the pain is really bad. The only down side for me is that the stimulator was placed on the left side for right sided pain and I've now developed TN on the right side. I'm fighting with this now, but it has given me some hope.

Complementary, Alternative and Natural Treatments

Complementary, Alternative and Natural Treatments

Complementary and Alternative Medicine (CAM) is the term for medical products, practices, and procedure that are not part of standard care. Standard care is what medical doctors, doctors of osteopathy and allied health professionals, such as nurses and physical therapists, practice. CAM is being used more widely and is becoming more acceptable in the conservative, medical community.

Complementary medicine can be used together with standard medical care. An example is acupuncture or medical Cannabis to help with side effects of cancer treatment or other illnesses.

Alternative medicine also can be used in place of standard medical care. An example is chelation therapy for heart disease, which seeks to remove excess metals from the blood, instead of using a standard approach.

We in no way discourage the use of natural and complementary treatment, but as with all treatments, we do encourage great care, research and a doctor's oversight. Some suggestions:

- Discuss any CAM treatments you are considering with your doctor because they may have side effects or interact with other medicines
- Find out what the research says about the CAM treatments you are considering.
- Choose CAM practitioners very carefully.
- Be choosy about which CAM treatments to try.
- Telling your doctor about any CAM and standard treatments you are considering, as well as doing lots of research on these treatments, is important because some natural and herbal compounds have serious interactions with medications and with each other. They may be detrimental to some medical

conditions and even cause fatal reactions. One good resource is the National Center for Complementary and Integrative Health (*nccih.nih.gov*).

As is often the case with TN, what may be helpful to one person may not be helpful to another person. It is important to be very careful and make wise decisions when deciding to use alternative, natural or complementary treatment methods. Read up on these methods, ask fellow TN support group members and always talk to your doctor. There are many specialists who practice in holistic medicine which include CAMs. They too are worth consideration and can prove to be a great help.

Acupuncture and Chiropractic

Wendy: Acupuncture helped calm the nervous system down for me. My acupuncturist was keenly aware that he could also amp the system up if not done properly. I found a different acupuncturist to help after he left town, and his work freed up the facial nerve so my left side of the mouth moves more, but more movement equals more pain. He also hurt me with a traditional chiropractic move. The work did not help my TN, which is actually TNP; instead, it created more TN pain.

Kiley Burns: Acupuncture actually gave me migraines.

Chiropractic and Upper Cervical Connection
National Upper Cervical Chiropractic Association

The upper cervical care under the tutelage of the National Upper Cervical Chiropractic Association (NUCCA) is a gentle, non-invasive technique of healing that can help restore body balance and good health. It was developed more than 40 years ago and focuses on the relationship between the upper cervical spine and its influence on the central nervous system and brain stem function. There are only approximately 2000 NUCCA chiropractors in the United States. For more information, visit *nucca.org*.

Disorders of the upper spine can cause TN and some people have found upper cervical chiropractic care to be helpful. This not a common cause, but is certainly worth checking into. It is advisable to get an X-ray and/or an MRI of the neck, if this seems to be a possible cause or factor of a person's trigeminal neuralgia.

As with all medical treatments, it is important to do your homework, as UCC is a very specialized treatment and requires extra training for the chiropractor. When looking for an upper cervical chiropractor, utilize the NUCCA website (*nucca.org*). Always shop around and if possible get recommendations from friends that have had upper cervical chiropractic treatments. A chiropractor not educated in upper spinal treatment can cause more harm.

Pam Whitling Elliott: I originally tried upper cervical chiropractic (UCC) care when I was first diagnosed, after I had heard of several people being pain free within several adjustments. I saw two doctors that used two different techniques, but they were not able to stop the pain, so I stopped going to them. While I did get a little relief, it wasn't enough to warrant continued visits after a year.

I also have atypical trigeminal neuralgia, which is much harder for the medical field to "fix," and I have never heard of UCC stopping the pain for this type of trigeminal neuralgia. Recently however, after I have had many medical procedures, the last two being an MVD and then nine months later they partially severed the trigeminal nerve, my pain in the first branch has gradually escalated, so I returned to UCC care to see if I could get any relief. It helped a lot this time. I am still in the first stages, but it's promising and if it continues to help, I hope to be able to lower my medications.

Supplements, Vitamins and Herbs

These are some of the supplements, vitamins, herbs and homeopathic tips that people have found helpful. Please be cautious, research and talk to your doctor before using alternative or complementary treatments.

Vitamins

- B COMPLEX
- Vitamin B12
- Vitamin B6
- Vitamin D
- Vitamin D3
- Vitamin K2
- CoQ10,
- Folic Acid
- Magnesium, 400mg per day
- Oil of Evening Primrose

Other

- Peppermint Oil: put on painful areas of face.
- Coconut Oil: swish in mouth for 20 minutes; helps with teeth pain.
- Liquid Magnesium: rub onto face, some report instant pain relief
- Fish Oil
- Krill Oil
- Horseradish or Hot Chinese Mustard: ingest, you may want to sit down when doing this one.
- Methyl B12, 5000 mcg: protects nerve tissue and brain cells; promotes better sleep and reduces toxic homocysteine to the essential amino acid methionine
- Melatonin: promotes a healthy night's sleep

- Horse Liniment: Absorbine Veterinary Liniment Gel, a topical analgesic available at Walmart
- Gallixa aka Gallium Maltolate: a compound cream worth discussing with your doctors
- Alpha Lipoic Acid in topical form
- Tart Cherries found in tablet form
- Colostrum Powder: to clean out microorganisms that can cause problems with the nerves
- Omega-3 plant oil (not fish)
- Try to eat natural, unprocessed foods like greens. Remember to eat the rainbow—a colorful diet.
- Don't forget warm Epsom salt baths.

It is important to say here that many with TN have chosen natural alternatives after trying and exhausting contemporary approaches. It's one of those things when you have tried so many medications and treatments that have failed, or have issues with intolerance of the medications, the more natural approaches may be a sufferer's only remaining option.

Medical Cannabis

The marijuana plant contains several chemicals that may prove useful for treating a range of illnesses or symptoms, leading many people to argue that it should be made legally available for medical purposes. In fact, a growing number of states (23 as of November 2014) have legalized marijuana's use for certain medical conditions. For more information, visit *mmj.org*.

Medical cannabis, or medical marijuana, refers to the use of cannabis and its constituent cannabinoids, such as tetrahydrocannabinol (THC) and cannabidiol (CBD), as medical therapy to treat disease or alleviate symptoms. There are many rare diseases and illnesses that may not respond well to conventional medicines, trigeminal neuralgia is one of these. THC and CBD together treat pain. THC stimulates appetite and reduces nausea, but it may also decrease pain, inflammation and spasticity. CBD is a non-psychoactive cannabinoid that may be useful in reducing pain and inflammation, controlling epileptic seizures and inhibiting cancer cell growth.

Medical Marijuana and Trigeminal Neuralgia

Once this topic was presented to the group, the response was overwhelming. Many people claim that medical marijuana helps more than conventional treatments and medications. Some people are from states where they can legally obtain medical marijuana, and some people live in non-legal states. Some have had medical marijuana recommended for their pain by their doctors.

Rebecca Webb: Does cannabis help? I have always wondered about that.

Betina Bach Knudsen: How do you injest Cannabis? Smoke, eat? Does it give you pain relief?

Kiley Burns: It's helping my mom and me. She takes the capsules and I smoke.

Dianna Vanderburg Demay: I saw the doctor on Saturday to get my medical marijuana license. (She is the same doctor that has been in the news about the young epileptic child and medical marijuana.) Unfortunately, my pain management doctor won't allow it, so I'm in a holding pattern right now. Thanks for the links; I'm doing all the research I can! Having TN-2 and AD with no surgical options and crazy meds, I'm getting *so* weary!

Alphonse Pellegrino: I have my legal medical marijuana license card for my glaucoma, but I also find great relief with it for my TN. It's the only time I feel like my old self; so I am self-medicating with a drug for one illness to help another. Before I was diagnosed, I use to drink alcohol to escape the pain, and since I have been on medications I have had maybe six drinks in the past year. Medical marijuana works on curbing the pain better than any pill I have taken; it makes me feel like the old me before trigeminal neuralgia—the happy-go-lucky guy that smiled all the time and not the miserable, sad and depressed person I am now.

Barbara McDoewll: I wish there was legal medical marijuana in Pennsylvania. I sometimes resort to drinking, not often, only when it is really bad and I happen to have some cash.

Kathy: I live in California and have had my medical marijuana license card for about four to five years. I use medical marijuana daily to relieve my trigeminal neuropathic pain. It at least helps me "zone out" for a few hours and not feel my pain. I either smoke or eat the edibles.

Dennis Gannon: Marijuana makes my trigeminal neuralgia and TMJ much worse, which in turn brings on migraines!

June Toland-Stephens: In my experience marijuana helps my TN-1 considerably, but some strains can aggravate my TN-2. I am for the rescheduling of cannabis as medically beneficial. I live in a non-legal state, so I cannot freely test different strains and different methods of use, such as oils and edibles.

How to Obtain a Medical Marijuana Card in Medically Legal States

- Find a physician: Some states have hundreds of physicians willing to write medical marijuana recommendations; some states have only a few. State medical marijuana laws and regulations vary by state.
- Find out if your condition is covered: Each state has a list of conditions that are approved for the use of medical marijuana. Check your state's listing to see

if you qualify. If you don't, learn whether or not you can submit a request for an exception.

- Understand your individual state's laws: Get a copy of the law and read it carefully. Each state's laws is different.

- Medical cannabis cards: Most states issue medical cannabis cards. First, patients must obtain a recommendation from a certified MD for legal medical marijuana based on ailments or sicknesses that the patient is experiencing. Upon approval by the doctor and the state, they are issued a medical cannabis card.

- Medical marijuana recommendation: Each state has different requirements and different conditions that are covered. A doctor experienced in recommending medical marijuana or your primary care physician may be able to help you obtain the needed recommendations.

- For more information, visit *mmj.org*.

Determine The Medical Marijuana Strain That's Right For You

Cannabis indica produces a higher level of CBD relative to THC. Indica is associated with sedative effects and is often preferred for nighttime use, including for treatment of insomnia. Indica is also associated with a more "stoned" or meditative sensation than the euphoric, stimulating effects of sativa. Indicas have elevated cannabinols showing more narcotic effects, stronger pain relievers and relaxing effects.

Cannabis sativa, on the other hand, produces a higher level of THC relative to CBD. Sativa is associated with a cerebral high and many patients experience stimulating effects. For this reason, sativa is often used for daytime treatment. It may cause more of a euphoric "high" sensation and tends to stimulate hunger. Sativa also exhibits a higher tendency to induce anxiety and paranoia, so patients prone to these effects may limit treatment with pure sativa or choose hybrid strains. For more information, visit *mmj.org*.

How TN Changes Our Lives

How TN Changes Our Lives

Simple little things that other people would never think about become major issues for people with trigeminal neuralgia. What things does TN keep you from doing that others are able to do normally?

LeeAnn Ryan: Playing in the snow with my son, like we use to do! I want to go outside, but I know that if I do, I will pay for it in a major way, very soon!

Rebecca Thorpe: Hair in my face. Some days, I just want to shave it off!

Sarah Edmondson: Eating food like subs or a big old cheeseburger! I have to cut up all my food and put it in the back of my mouth to eat because biting into food is way too painful. Also, talking and singing; I use to love doing karaoke and can't anymore because how are you going to sing a song when you have to stop for 15 seconds while having an attack? I used to love the snow, but now the wind and cold are so difficult. I want to be able to take my kids sledding when they're old enough.

Suzi Strand: Eating, sleeping and playing music are what I miss the most. I was a classical oboist before TN entered my life. I even sat in and played with the Boston Pops Orchestra. Unfortunately, my facial pain won't let me play musical instruments that touch my face anymore. I have to avoid concerts, loud music and movie theaters, all of which are a struggle and triggers for me.

Alphonse Pellegrino: Shaving every day is something I no longer am able to do. I only shave once a week, unless I have to go out.

Pauline Donye: I am no longer able to use my electric toothbrush; I can only use it on the right side and then brush *very* carefully with an ordinary brush on the left. Sometimes I can't chew properly, and I end up swallowing bigger pieces of food than normal. I'm always afraid my teeth or breath smell. When I am going out shopping alone I'm always afraid of a crisis so I drag my son with me in case I need help. I nearly choked on a small piece of chicken from chicken soup—I could not chew properly because of the pain. I have lost all confidence. I'm afraid to go to the bank alone, not just because the pain might come on, but because I spend so much time at home that I feel like I am useless outside of the home.

Our Relationships
The Supportive and Un-supportive

Our relationships with our loved ones can be our strongest support or it can devastate us when the relationship goes bad because of trigeminal neuralgia. Unfortunately, people judge others by what they see and often conclude a person can or cannot do something by the way they look. Like with other hidden illnesses, our limitations and struggles are not often believed. At one point or another, most of us have been accused of faking, being lazy, seeking drugs and making up excuses to get out of things.

It is very difficult to explain at times what TN is to our family and friends; to explain what occurs or how it feels when we experience a flare; or to try and explain why or how we are in a constant flux of pain. Many times we don't understand it ourselves. To some people it may appear as though we are making excuses to avoid activities like birthdays, celebrations, holidays or events, and as time goes by our family and friends often stop extending the invitations altogether.

Many medical professionals along with our family and friends are misinformed about opiates, believing they never work on TN and/or neuropathic pain, and many loved ones have deduced that the TN sufferer is a drug addict. Many family and friends believe their loved one is just seeking attention or that it's all in their head. This is especially true when many doctors wrongly think the same way.

One hope for this book is that when family and friends read the stories of other TN sufferers, their perspective about TN will change and they will be more understanding and compassionate with their loved one who has TN.

Many TN suffers have lost relationships with family members, friends and loved ones. People who don't have TN just can't believe that it can be that painful. How does one describe the worst pain on earth? In stark contrast, are the husbands and wives, children and parents, friends and loved ones who give us strength every day to fight this beast. Our supportive loved ones may never know how many times they have helped save us from totally giving up! We understand our illness hurts you also. Hats off and much respect to all of you that have helped, stood by and supported your loved one with trigeminal neuralgia. Thank You!

How TN Affects Our Relationships

Kathy: This is one area that is very sensitive to me, and I am sure I am not the only person who feels that way. Since getting trigeminal neuralgia in 2004, I no longer have the desire to make new friends because each friend I have made since getting sick has abandoned me for various reasons. One "friend" thought I was in too much pain from a swollen leg and therefore she thought I was too "drugged up" and I couldn't feel the pain because I was taking medication for my trigeminal neuralgia. She then proceeded to tell me I should, "get help with my drug problem." She clearly did not understand the depths of trigeminal neuralgia and what she "felt and thought" was entirely different from what I was actually feeling and going through!

Then there were my trigeminal neuralgia friends, and we discussed the importance of sticking together and not abandoning one another, but these friends have also left. I occasionally correspond via email with another TN friend.

The loss that hurt me the most is that of my sister. My three brothers have stuck by my side, but not my sister—the one person who is supposed to be your best friend! We grew up together, played together, shared a bedroom and told secrets to each other. The bond we had growing up, even when we were arguing, was undeniable. When I was first ill, I recall her telling our parents, "That's my sister. I'm so worried about her." After about three years, my sister chose not to believe in trigeminal neuralgia and my illness. Why? Because I take pain medication! She chose to believe instead that I was a drug seeker. Never a day in my life have I taken any drugs or alcohol in excess! Sure, I partied in my younger years, but who didn't? It hurts me to the core of my soul when I see other sisters on social media supporting their ill sisters. As sisters, we should have been able to work through this. Maybe one day she will be the supportive sister I crave.

My biggest supporters have been my son, my parents, my brothers, my sister-in-law, my BFF (you know who you are) and my extended family! And honestly, if it were not for them, I would not be here today. It would take this entire book for me to relate all the wonderful and supportive ways they have been there for me since my getting TN. I feel very blessed to have them in my life! I have one true friend that has always been there for me since we were 14 years old. We've been through everything together! She lives in Washington and I'm in California. I see her one to two times per year and maybe the distance is why she is still in my life and hasn't left yet! There you have it, my story of lost family and friends, all because of an illness that doesn't have a cure and entered my life in the blink of an eye; not something I or anyone else ever asked for or deserved!

Christy Ritter: My husband supports and stands up for me a lot, even when it's against his own family, because I can't without causing me even more stress and pain. He has been even more understanding since the pain is now full blown and constant. I know it also puts a big strain on him, working extra hard to pay my medical bills, taking care of me, helping with the girls and housework. He's been great!

Pam Whitling Elliott: My three adult daughters and one adult son who have families of their own have been very supportive of my illness. A couple of my daughters help take me to doctor appointments when and if they can. Most of my family is now supportive. At first, some didn't understand, maybe they still don't, but the ones that matter the most do understand and it has been very difficult for them. They see me struggle and suffer every day. Some days are terrible and they get frustrated because they want me "fixed", but there is no fixing atypical TN. My husband has the most stress, but he doesn't complain. He accepts it and reminds me of our wedding vows—for better or worse, in sickness and in health. He asks me, "What if I had TN? Would you do the same for me?" It keeps it in perspective because his work load is sometimes so heavy. When I can't do the shopping, extra cleaning, cooking or even bring in the mail, it adds an extra burden on him. I couldn't do this without his support, help and understanding.

Mark Steadman: Everything changes. Our families have had to adapt to the illness and we have all missed out on so much, including visits and family activities. Our families see us at our worst when you just want to hide away. I'm lucky that I have been pain-free since my MVD, but my family and I lost four years of our lives to TN. I honestly wouldn't have survived this without my family to pick me up.

Dating and Being Single with TN

Alphonse Pellegrino asks: Why does having trigeminal neuralgia and being single make a person want to date, but also not want to date?

Some people with trigeminal neuralgia and other chronic illnesses avoid dating altogether for fear of becoming a burden to other people. People often assume that their illness or situation is the only thing that prospective partners or friends will notice about them or that is what you need to tell them first thing. But that is untrue. The rest of the world sees the entire package. Don't give up on dating yet. For one reason or another, we are all difficult to date.

Allison Ramirez: I'm answering because I was single for 16 years after my marriage failed. I'm not single anymore, and I met my husband long after I got atypical trigeminal neuralgia. He knew from the beginning that I had multiple painful neurological conditions that are incurable and make me unreliable as far as planning anything. I had several prior relationships fall apart because the other person could not handle being with someone in pain all the time. They resented the fact that I never knew how I was going to feel at any given time and couldn't handle the emotional roller coaster we were on. I just wanted to let you know that there are people out there who are willing and able to be with someone with this condition.

Alphonse Pellegrino: I am interested in meeting somebody and starting a relationship because I believe it would help with being depressed, but I also believe it would be ideal to be in a relationship with another person who has trigeminal neuralgia. Who better to understand what we deal with and to be supportive of each other? I'm tired of being alone, but also don't know if it is fair to drag someone into the hellish life of trigeminal neuralgia, so I believe a single's group like this would be a good way to find others with TN who might like to meet.

In 2014, Alphonse Pellegrino started a Trigeminal Neuralgia Singles of the World Facebook group. There are only two requirements: You must have trigeminal neuralgia and/or facial pain, and you must be single. To join, type "Trigeminal Neuralgia Single's of the World" in the Facebook search bar.

Our Mates

Whether you are married or dating, male or female, your TN or other major disability will have an impact on your mate. The guilt we feel is heavy! Many people that suffer with TN have lost their mates, spouses, boyfriends, girlfriends and other loved ones because of TN. For better or worse, but what about if it *is* the worst?

Lisa Malecha: Due to my three surgeries, all of the doctors' appointments and taking care of me, my husband ended up losing his job. My daughter became the mother figure in our house. It didn't really affect our son. My mom, dad and my two brothers had all these expectations of me (showing up for holidays, birthdays and other family events) that I just could not meet all the time, and that wasn't good enough for them. They said that it was my choice to distance myself from the family. I did the best I could day by day. They have chosen to not be part of my life or my kids' lives. I feel it's easier for them to distance themselves from me than to have to deal with this disease and all of its effects.

June Toland-Stephens: When my husband and I first got together, he handed me his disability award notice and had me read everything that was wrong with him. He then asked me if I thought I could love him. I knew I already did, but I remember thinking to myself: Yes, but no amount of paperwork can explain all of my disabilities, and can you love me? I honestly didn't believe he would stick with me. But he has for almost 10 years now. He has learned about TN from me, but since I started writing this book, he has joined a couple of support groups and has learned from many. He held me up in writing this book, sometimes calming me down and other times spurring me on. Thank you dear. I love you.

Sex and TN

No more lovers' kisses so sweet and tender. They have become stabs of daggers. No more soft caress of the cheek. Now it feels like claws ripping at the flesh. The desire for pleasure gets overpowered by the intensity of our pain. The medications can make the libido shrink, hide or die. But more than just the sex act, it can sap the romance and enjoyment right out of the relationship. The sadness tears us apart and no doubt puts a strain on our relationships with our mates. And that affects the sex life in return. Talking about it and even therapy may be the answer for some. One of the most supportive things a mate can give to a person with trigeminal neuralgia or any disability is patience and understanding.

Barbara McDowell: My relationship with my husband is very strained at times. I think he gets frustrated that we do not have sex often because of atypical trigeminal neuralgia and arthritis pain. For the most part, he is great and understands how I am feeling. I think it just gets to him sometimes; it's frustrating and I don't know what to do to fix it. When I am in a lot of pain, I just want to be left alone.

Betsy Taylor Alexander: Everything from kissing and face caresses to sex could set off my trigeminal neuralgia. But sometimes it doesn't. I have been married for 32 years to a wonderful man and not being able to kiss each other when we want is horrible. The intimacy we have lost, in addition to the loss to the rest of our lives, makes me very sad and just makes me cry.

Betina Bach Knudsen: When I'm in pain, that's all I can focus on, and I try to hide it from my boyfriend, but he notices it right away. He feels like he is hurting me, and I tend to lose focus. I am now using improved medication, and I'm practically pain-free for now, so a sex life is again possible. But there are a lot of side effects from the medication, and they affect my mood and energy levels, which also affect my sex life.

Dianna Vanderburg Demay: This thread is making me weep. I also have anesthesia dolorosa (half my face is numb), and I have said since day one what I miss the most is my husband's kisses—that communication and connection of two souls melting together, even if you're standing in the kitchen. So sad! Now, 10 to 11 years later, trigeminal neuropathic pain and anesthesia dolorosa have destroyed so much, but still the thing I miss the most is the feel of my husband's kisses.

Let's save the face so we can kiss our mates.

A Kiss
by Allison Ramirez

How can such a gentle touch
A kiss
A sweet caress
Become such pain

Once I welcomed the feel
Of my lover's hand
His lips upon mine
The gentle closeness of love

Pain has taken the place
Of the joy
Of the unexpected kiss
The gentle caress of my face

Inwardly I cringe in fear
Hoping he doesn't see
The dread I hide
When he comes near

Will his touch cause me pain
Will his kisses sear
Send burning waves
Shocking stabs
Stinging zaps
Across my face

The unseen cost
Of love and affection
The fear
The dread
The inconsolable sadness
Of what I have lost
The pain I hide

Parenting with Trigeminal Neuralgia

Christy Ritter: This one is really hard for me. My kids are 7 and 3 years old. My oldest child remembers me before the pain took over. We used to do a lot of things together and play a lot. Now I am not able to play with my children because the pain is constant. She will cry sometimes saying she wants her mommy back. Well, I want her mommy back too! My youngest doesn't quite get it, but she *knows* she can't touch my face. Lately I've been stuck in bed due to all the pain, and I hear them playing or watching TV knowing they are alone. It breaks my heart; I used to be such a good mommy. Sometimes I think it would be better if I wasn't around. I *hate* this!

Suzi Strand: The momma guilt gets to me a lot. Lately I've been having a hard time with all of my illnesses, so I've been spending more time lying down. I can hear my kids playing and talking, and every fiber of my being wants to go hang out with them, but sometimes I just can't and I lie in bed and cry!

Kristi Leeder: My children have never known me when I was pain-free. I want to play in the snow with them and just do fun, regular activities with my children that normal parents do with their children.

Our Family, Friends and Caregivers
A Caregivers Perspective

The following is an insightful interview with Matt Williams, caregiver to Sheri Neumoyer.

How long have you been Sheri's caregiver?

Sheri had her first microvascular decompression (MVD) about five years ago in 2009, and I effectively became her caregiver after that surgery failed. I had helped her before that, but her first MVD really took away most of the self-sufficiency she had managed to hold onto. Because her second MVD followed the first one by only a handful of weeks, it was a destructive procedure and gave her severe dysaesthesia, on top of her TN, and she ended up immobile for a while.

Had you heard of TN before meeting Sheri?

I had never heard of TN before.

Did you know her before she got trigeminal neuralgia?

Sheri and I actually met before her trigeminal neuralgia onset, and she started casually following an online journal I kept. We had a number of mutual friends and had both been part of the same performing group, though not simultaneously.

I understand you attend appointments with Sheri and have been with her through different procedures. What advice would you give to other TN caregivers?

Doctors' appointments have a few caveats for someone taking medicines that impair short-term memory, such as anticonvulsants. We discuss beforehand what she plans to address with the doctor, so that I can jog her memory and provide some prompting, if needed. I will often supplement her comments to the doctor with my own observations. I bring a written list of her questions for the doctor and take notes on her behalf in order to let her focus on what the doctor is saying. Before the end of the appointment, I will recapitulate what has happened to help her recall if there were any other topics she needed to bring up. Afterwards, I have my written notes to review with her; she often has incomplete or sparse recall of the doctor's visit and reviewing the notes also helps her remember details that would otherwise be fleeting.

I know her medications and most of her medical history, so I am able to fill in the gaps for her as well as aid with paperwork. Before she signs anything critical, I read over it, provide a summary and answer her questions. I try to anticipate any concerns she might have so that she can formulate questions from her thoughts should they become jumbled. This also extends to proofreading the things she writes. Sheri is quite brilliant and expressive, but her confusion from the pain and the medications often results in writing that looks like it was written by someone while falling asleep.

This also helps her feel more comfortable writing to her friends online because it's extremely rare that she gets out to socialize. Often she is unable to talk on the phone so communicating with friends online via her smart phone is usually the extent of her social life. Prior to having TN she used to love to write, now she will produce something poetic, but leave out a critical word or she will produce a keen observation, but punctuate it bizarrely. Having someone to help her write to her friends is helpful because she's already a recluse, frustrated by her inabilities.

We have realized that it is important for a caregiver to monitor the self-esteem of their charge, especially when that person is afflicted by such an overwhelming and debilitating condition at a young age. It's dangerously easy for someone in Sheri's situation to begin feeling robbed of a large extent of her life. It does not behoove her to feel embarrassed or isolated as well!

It may sound like I do a lot as a caregiver, and I have been very fortunate to have the time and ability to be so involved in her life, but it is my belief that someone with an illness that intensely affects nearly every facet of one's life may benefit from assistance distributed broadly over many categories. Sheri is my friend as well, but my function as a caregiver is independent of that. In fact, if I thought of her as a friend merely in need of various forms of aid, I would likely grow tired of helping her. I am not merely trying to go the extra mile because she is also my friend; I do what I do because I am the caregiver for a fellow human who needs all the help she can get to deal with her illness. In fact, I want to mention something we have observed as her list of good friends has dwindled over the years. Separating who she is as a person from how she is affected by her illness is absolutely vital for anyone who has remained in her life.

Individuals that have failed to comprehend that Sheri has a devastating, invisible illness eventually walk away. Some may be able to parrot back a list of ways that Sheri's life has been trampled upon by TN, yet still not realize that TN is not a personality trait that she maintains. An intractable illness is not like an article of clothing that can be removed, nor like a bandage that can be discarded when it has served its purpose. People with TN didn't elect to have such an alienating condition, even if the time of onset seems in retrospect to have been under their control, which it rarely is.

Any person who becomes a caregiver has to bear these things in mind, lest one run out of patience.

Brian Malecha

The following is a husband's struggle with his wife's trigeminal neuralgia.

The simple truth is that TN hurts all of those that live with or have a close relationship with the TN sufferer. In Lisa's case, it has taken away how she wanted to be a mother. It has changed the way she approaches life and thus has changed the way I approach life. Medical costs and the constant discomfort took away dreams of family vacations, and date nights become non-existent when your date for the night feels self-conscious about eating out in public.

Both of your lives become consumed by TN. You watch as the relationships with your extended family and friends from the old days wither up and die when you can't make this party or that barbecue because it is a bad pain day. You watch your daughter be embarrassed at a softball game when a teammate assumes her parents are divorced because her mom never shows up. You feel alone because you attend events with the kids and end up going alone, while your TN afflicted partner is home alone struggling with pain. You struggle with the work/home balance because of the bad days and the need to help, comfort, and care for your TN spouse. Even the most understanding of bosses gets tired of you missing work to help take care of a grown adult. Your relationship becomes more of a caretaker and patient than husband and wife. The hurt we feel as a loved one is not the intense physical pain that you feel, but it is a hurt nonetheless.

I feel that as a country we seem to spend a large amount of money on medications and treating symptoms and not nearly enough on prevention and cures.

Caregiving Tips from a Caring Mom

Below are Michele's practical tips to help prepare and adjust to the new role as a caregiver.

It is important to learn the proper name of your child's illness.

It is important to educate yourself as much as possible about your child's illness. Use the computer, social media and library; attend support group meetings, etc.

Know that good friends and even other family members will not understand many things about this illness, like medications, the many doctors involved, why the patient does not look sick (usually), canceled plans, and more.

Your child may not be able to go out in the evenings as pain levels tend to get worse as the day goes on.

When possible, attend your adult child's doctor appointments, tests and scans. Having a hand to hold during these difficult times is very comforting. When the doctor is speaking, four ears are better than two and this allows the caregiver to take notes while the patient is listening to the doctor.

When possible, go to the seminars, support group meetings and conferences, etc. as this will help the caregiver, support person, friends and family members to become more informed about the illness.

Encourage your child to search out and attend local support group meetings. Many support groups are happy to include caregivers at their meetings.

Go on social media, you would be amazed that there are so many people out there that have the same illness; the support for both the ill child and the caregiver is amazing!

Be realistic and honest with your ill child. Don't tell them what they want to hear. Tell them the truth, however difficult it may be.

Our Social Lives

June Toland-Stephens: As TN takes over our lives, we by nature tend to isolate ourselves from others. Many of us spend our social life in TN support groups and have very little interaction with non-trigeminal neuralgia friends. Many times, we can't explain to others what is going on, and the truth is we often don't understand it ourselves; it would take weeks to explain it and trying to get someone else to understand why we have all these strange issues is extremely difficult. Often we find ourselves starting to explain TN and at first they are interested, but not many want to listen to a long, depressing explanation full of medical terms.

Betsy Taylor Alexander: I have no social life left. I am not who I used to be, and it has affected my relationships with friends. I have one friend that I have had since first grade and of course she has stuck by me—even stayed up at the hospital for a while so my husband could get out for a couple of hours. I feel like people just don't know how to treat me . . . too much pity. First question that I usually hear is, how am I doing, but it's said in such a way that makes me feel like I have two heads and six arms, like I am a freak.

Barbara McDowell: My social life was never busy, but I have found that it has gotten worse. Sometimes I can't go out because the pain is so bad. Sometimes I go out anyway and then pay dearly when I get home. I do *not* want to spend my life all alone. Heck, I have a great nephew I have not met yet because every time I think I will go visit, either the beast rears its ugly head or I get arthritis so bad, and every once in a while, it is a combination of both.

Suzi Strand: Facebook allows me to at least feel like I have a social life.

Kathy: I had a wonderful social life before trigeminal neuralgia entered my life. Now I have nothing—no more holidays, birthdays, special occasions, and celebrating with my family. My pain is so extreme, and as the day progresses so does my pain. By 3:30 p.m. every single day, I am in bed, bundled up with a heating pad, scarf, heated mattress pad, anything I can do to keep my face warm and out of pain. What kind of life is that? I tell you, that's no way to live. I am merely existing!

Mental Health Care and TN

Mental Health Care and TN

TN, like other major illnesses, causes depression, anxiety, PTSD and many other mental ailments. Some TN sufferers may have mental health problems that worsen their TN, even if those problems are not related to their TN. In both cases good mental health care can make a world of difference.

June Toland-Stephens: The only way I have found to explain how it mentally feels to be tormented by TN is to compare it to POWs. We are tortured, with shocks to our heads. We fear of the smallest things—a breeze, a kiss, or touch. Many sufferers isolate themselves. The anxiety and PTSD a trigeminal neuralgia sufferer experiences is enhanced and complicated. The fear of triggers, flares and attacks can be as crippling as the pain. Post-traumatic stress in TN is not "post"; it's ever-present.

Jenny LeCompte: I know I've seen somewhere that PTSD symptoms can be caused by chronic pain and seriously I feel a difference between my trauma-driven PTSD and what I absolutely feel is PTSD related directly to my trigeminal neuralgia. I have serious anxiety over the dumbest things, like even opening the door to go outside and feeling that gust of wind or having the sun on my face ... *at all*. I have serious anxiety over anyone asking me to do anything, like hanging out or making plans, which I guess I'm fortunate, no one asks me anymore because I'm always afraid I will have to cancel and deal with their judgment. Let's face it, we're all afraid of the dentist not just because of the fear normal people have, but because of our TN.

Kiley Burns: I was diagnosed with depression and anxiety when I was 15 years old, but of course it was worsened by my TN diagnosis. I have an excellent psychiatrist who handles my medications, acts as a kind of a counselor when I need to vent and also treats my mom, so she knows my background and hers very well.

June Toland-Stephens: My diagnoses after my TN and close call with suicide was PTSD, depression and, my favorite, "failure to adapt to my disabilities." It is my firm belief that most people with TN can benefit from some type of mental health counseling. However, this is where we face many hurdles. Many people with TN. have been told the pain is in their head and that tends to turn people away from counselors.

Kathy: It was about four years into my illness when one day my dad said to me, "The life you once knew is now gone." That was honesty and something that my dad needed to say, and it was just the jolt I needed to jump-start my new life!

It is a difficult challenge to find a counselor that has even a little bit of TN knowledge. The key is to find a counselor that works for you. Don't be afraid to look for another one if the current counselor isn't working for you.

Support groups are another great option to obtain the support you are looking for, whether it is through a local support group or online/social media. Over the last few years, many support groups have been started online on Facebook, Twitter and many other forums. In these groups, we have found patience, support, understanding and so much more! Most people in the online support groups have never met one other person with TN in real life. However, those we have met on social media and online are often closer to us than our real-life friends and family. Only another person with TN can truly understand the pain and fears we go through.

Post-Nerve Resection Thoughts

by Sheri Lyn Neumoyer
August 2009

There's a silent monster you cannot see.
It's capable of things no one believes.
I wake in the morning with the sun so bright.
Then it bursts through my face with its venomous bite.

I reach for my bottles to poison this beast,
As it eats at my face as if it's a feast.
I cry, but I can no longer feel my tears.
My face is dead now I chose to kill my face in hopes
to kill the monster.

But the monster lives on, lives on to torture me.
I wish I knew why you are punishing me?
I want to keep fighting but where do I find the will?
Most of the time I find it in a bottle, a bottle filled with pills.

I swallow them with hope, and then I wait.
I never know if they'll help, if they'll make me stupid,
weary or just pass out.
I'm so tired I don't want to fight anymore.
I sit silently and look out my window.

The green grass is so pretty.
Why won't you let me go outside?
I'm just going through the motions of existing.
I just exist to be in pain.

What kind of life is that?
It's not a life. It's just not a life at all.
It feels like I've lost everything,
Everything I've ever known.

The Suicide Disease

Trigeminal neuralgia has been dubbed The Suicide Disease. There are many people that do not like this nickname and would like to do away with it, but the fact remains that extreme pain from TN or other very painful conditions can and have driven people to the brink of suicide and very sadly, some have taken their lives.

June Toland-Stephens: My close call with suicide came after yet another visit to a neurosurgeon in the hope of finding relief. When the surgeon said, "It sounds like trigeminal neuralgia, but it's so rare I doubt the diagnosis," I could handle that. I had already gotten used to hearing: it is, it isn't, it's too rare, it just can't be, but when he added, "Even if it is trigeminal neuralgia, I don't think we can help you," it was like he jerked the carpet of hope right out from under me. I left the office nearly hysterical.

The surgeon's office was on a busy street in a big city, next to the hospital. I stood on the curb and my thoughts went something like this: "I can't take this pain anymore and no one can help me. I just can't endure it anymore." Realize that I was 39 years old and had suffered a long, long time. I decided I was going to wait for a big truck and step in front of it. I didn't want anyone to know what I had done and planned for it to look like an accident. As I stood there I mentally went through my list of loved ones, my daughter, my two sons, they were grown and it was for them that I wanted it to look like an accident, but when I came to my sweet little granddaughter, at that time my only grandchild, I took a step back and that's when I knew no matter how bad the pain or what I suffer, there are still things in life worth living for. Thank you baby Rose, you will someday know you saved your grandma's life. (I have written this in tears.)

Suzi Strand: I remember the night the thought of living in this constant pain was too much. I wanted to end my suffering, but I didn't want my children to be left to find me. I reached out to someone I had been chatting with on Facebook who dealt with chronic pain. He stayed up with me all night and talked. I felt a lot less alone in my struggle and

I learned a lot of new coping skills along the way, which have helped transform me into someone who enjoys each day—not everything in the day, but every day I find something to be thankful for, and that helps get me to tomorrow.

Sarah Edmondson: So the thought of death has crossed my mind. I think things like, "I don't want to live if this is the rest of my life." It is so hard to keep going after you've lost the life you once knew and lose your dreams because they no longer seem feasible. Though I have thought I wanted to die, I just could never see myself taking my own life. Someone would have to find me and no one deserves that. It just feels like such a selfish decision, and selfish I am not. And even though I say that, I understand 100 percent why people do it, especially being in pain like this. What did people do before modern medicine? To live forever in pain with no relief, I would probably drink myself to death or something, that's such a scary thought. This disease makes you lose hope and without hope you spend every day fighting to find the reasons to stay alive and to keep going.

Rebecca Webb: Yes I have thought of it because the pain is indescribable. It just drains everything out of you, and I don't have anything left. But I have not tried suicide because I have kids and I want to be here for them. Most of the time, I want someone to break my jaw. And you can use my name; I'm not ashamed of these monsters.

Kathy: I can honestly say that when my pain gets so bad and extreme and when I think about what my future holds, I have thought about suicide. If my future is anything like these past 10 years have been like, I wonder if I can truly I make it. The main reason I'm still here is my family and my son. I could never leave them!

Mike Gaubert: When I had the first severe pain episodes in my temple area, I thought about suicide for six seconds; I thought of taking my gun, putting it to my head and pulling the trigger. But then I thought of the love of Jesus Christ and His love for me, and that gave me strength.

The support groups we have formed are our group therapy. And many of us have sat up all night chatting online with someone on the edge. The peer counseling in the Facebook TN support groups is amazing—24 hours a day, 7 days a week, 365 days a year there is always someone in one of the groups to listen and help. We've seen new members come in suicidal and gain the strength to not only fight on for themselves, but also become advocates for all TN sufferers. We cannot overstate how important it is to have a crisis plan and to have a person or persons we can turn to when these dark times come.

It's hard to be positive when so much negative is happening to you and your loved ones. Never blame yourself for what you cannot control. Allow yourself to be weak. Sometimes we just need a good cry and a good friend.

June Toland-Stephens: The group I started, which led to this book, has grown to over 1,300 members as of this writing. It's a wonderful place to find support and learn more about living with TN. There are many good groups that serve different needs. We have included an appendix with many support groups and organizations where you can find help. If you feel you may harm yourself. Go to the emergency room or call a suicide hotline. And know that 24/7, 365 days a year there are many other TN brothers and sisters on Facebook, Twitter and many other places that will listen and understand.

Hope

Hope

Words on Hope
by Wendy
July 15, 2014

I live in hope. I live in pain, chronic, intractable pain. Since November 1999, I've been in mind-numbing, spirit-killing pain. There are so many things that I used to take for granted, that everyone takes for granted, that I can no longer do . . . and yet I also live in hope.

Surely I have my ups and downs. One of the things I can no longer do, without paying for it in excruciating pain, is smiling. Yet the absence of smiling is not the same as the absence of joy, even if it looks like it. People closest to you can be trained to know this if they are willing; they aren't always willing. This is where hope comes in. Like a bad country song, I've been at bottom only to find that bottom falls out and there is another low. And still, I have held on to hope. It is a core of my being.

Many people facing a devastating disease such as TN are confused and lose all sense of hope somewhere in the midst of medication, surgery and seeking a "fix" for the pain. At this point in time these are really only temporary fixes that do work on some people for longer or shorter lengths of time (20 years or 2 months, depending on a host of issues). It is very easy to lose one's sense of self and sense of hope, to give one's self over to this dis-ease, but hope (among other things) can guide the way.

Without hope, I would not be getting out of bed in the morning or staying out of bed for the day. Hope gets me up and keeps me going, as much as I go anymore. (TN has taken me from a mover and shaker "get 'er done" kind of person, to a person who has come to terms with the "being" side of life. I've also learned to appreciate naps.) Hope is what keeps me sane when the pain feels like something gripping deep into my face and behind my eye (or wherever it turns up in its traditional TN, branch 2 pattern), stabbing, slashing and burning.

What do I hope for? I hope that the pain will lessen and sometimes it does. I hope for understanding and awareness and set about to educate and build awareness when I feel up to it. I hope for better treatment at the doctors' offices and for better treatments for the pain. And, most audaciously of all, I hope for a cure.

For many years, a cure was not even on the horizon, but now, thanks to the Facial Pain Research Foundation, I can see a cure or cures coming within my lifetime – and something that might even help me!

Hope based on solid fact's, growing closer every day. Now that is something worth helping to make come to fruition, certainly something worth hoping for, and something that makes it easier to bear this relentless pain. The promise that it won't be forever!

June Toland-Stephens: Having tried countless medications, procedures and brain surgeries with the pain ending up just as bad or worse, has caused many of us to lose our hope. Many had given up on ever finding an answer. Many of us have stopped going to doctors about our TN. Once a doctor I was seeing for something else asked me what I do for my TN. I looked him straight in the face and without missing a beat said, "Suffer, I suffer." When I learned about the great strides the Facial Pain Research Foundation was making, my thought and I'm sure so many others' also was: "Finally there is HOPE!"

Hope
by June Toland-Stephens

We hope to feel the sweet joy of a cool breeze across our cheeks and not fear or flinch.

We hope to kiss our mates and children with no fear of pain.

We hope that our young children with TN won't have to endure repeated brain surgeries.

We hope that not one more person with TN will be told they are crazy or a drug seeker.

We hope for better education for those that treat us, as it is so desperately needed.

We hope that in telling our stories and sharing our experiences, we can paint a bigger picture and expose the beast we call TN.

We hope to have our lives back, our families back—to be able to be the parent, spouse, mate, friend and person that TN has robbed us from being.

We hope to live without the extreme, intense pain and with the equally debilitating fear of pain.

We hope for a cure.

Our Hope Is In Research.

Our hope is in The Facial Pain Research Foundation and the researchers. The Foundation is amazing and the success of the mouse stem cell model is already a major breakthrough. They have restored our hope.

June Toland: While on a Greyhound bus going through the middle of nowhere, I went online and read about the success of the stem cell mouse model. I'm sure some people on the bus thought I was crazy when I sang out, "The mouse model worked! The mouse model worked! The mouse model worked!"

The DNA study to find the genetic marker(s) may help us find what predisposes a person to TN. Knowing this could not only impact TN sufferers. What are the possibilities that it's the same DNA marker in other neuro-pain conditions?

The Myelin study seeks to find out answers about myelin repair. The recently published findings are amazing. These and other studies being done at the Foundation each approach finding a cure from a different angle and yet work together as a whole toward one goal: *a cure*!

Thank you to all who work for The Facial Pain Research Foundation and an extra special thank you and much gratitude to each of the researchers and their teams. No amount of words, even if we wrote a thousand books, could ever tell how much hope you have given us.

A cure for trigeminal neuralgia, this is our hope! Beyond hope for TN sufferers, these studies go way beyond TN or facial pain. The studies will have wide application to many types of neural pain. Hope not just for us TNers. Hope for a world in pain.

Hope

by Allison Ramirez
January 27, 2015

I had a dream slumbering in the night
A dream where this pain has ended
A dream I hold so tight
A dream I am mended

I want my dream to come true
This dream of health and vigor
A dream so many hold on to
A dream that life is bigger

Bigger than this constant pain
That endlessly wears me down
Worrying me until I feel insane
And I wear a constant frown

I dream a cure is found
For these damaged nerves
That I wear smiles all around
Face life with renewed verve

Healing and strength will be found
This dream I have will come true
We can stand on solid ground
This I wish for you and me

Organizations, Support Groups and Resources

TN Organizations

Facial Pain Research Foundation
facingfacialpain.org

The Facial Pain Association, formerly The Trigeminal Neuralgia Association
fpa-support.org

Trigeminal Neuralgia Association UK
tna.org.uk

Canadian Trigeminal Neuralgia Association, Toronto/York Region group
catna2.ca

International Trigeminal Neuralgia and Me
TNnME.com

Facebook Support Groups

Trigeminal Neuralgia & Facial Pain
Trigeminal Neuralgia Support
Trigeminal Neuralgia Family
Trigeminal Neuralgia Help Group
Trigeminal Neuralgia -- The UK's TN Facebook Group
Trigeminal Neuralgia (TN) UK
End Trigeminal Neuralgia
https://www.facebook.com/endTrigeminalNeuralgia
Trigeminal Neuralgia Sufferers and Supporters
Trigeminal Neuralgia Support Group Ireland
Trigeminal Neuralgia Support & Care UK

Trigeminal Neuralgia - Facial Pain
Stop Trigeminal Neuralgia and Charcot Marie Tooth
NC Trigeminal Neuralgia Support
Geniculate Neuralgia
Young Adults with Trigeminal Neuralgia
TNnME News and Media
TN advocates
Trigeminal Neuralgia Eastern States
MVD Patient Support
Neuropathic - Nerve Pain Support Group
Trigeminal Neuralgia & Social Security (SSI, & SSD)
Trigeminal Neuralgia Support India
Hemifacial Spasm International Support Group
Natural Approach to Trigeminal Neuralgia
NEURALGIA CENTRAL
Light Up Teal for Trigeminal Neuralgia
Occipital Neuralgia
Struggle and Strength - TN Inspired Art
Surgical Options for Head and Facial Pain Support Group
TN, ATN, ON Sufferers Group
Trigeminal Neuralgia - The UK's TN facebook group
NEURALGIA DO TRIGÊMEO BRASIL
Missouri Trigeminal Neuralgia
Occipital Neuralgia Support Group
Dedicated to Trigeminal Neuralgia and other chronic illness warriors!
Occipital and Peripheral Nerve Stimulation
CHRISTIANS WITH CHRONIC POLYNEURALGIC PAIN
Migraine or Occipital Neuralgia
The Cluster Headache Support Group
Faith Based Trigeminal Neuralgia & Chronic Pain Support Group
Young Adults with Trigeminal Neuralgia

TN Recipes
Our Neuropathy Friends
NEURALGIA DO TRIGÊMIO A NOSSA DOR
Trigeminal Neuralgia Awareness Fighters
Trigeminal Neuralgia Mental Health Brothers And Sisters
Trigeminal Neuralgia Friends & Family
Trigeminal Neuralgia Association of Canada
Dedicated to Trigeminal Neuralgia and other chronic illness warriors!

Non-Facebook Online Support Groups

livingwithtn.org
dailystrength.org/c/Trigeminal-Neuralgia/support-group
neurotalk.psychcentral.com/forum26.html

Other Helpful Resources

Trigeminal neuralgia fact sheet from National Institute of Health
ninds.nih.gov/disorders/trigeminal_neuralgia/detail_trigeminal_neuralgia.htm

Occipital Neuralgia/American Association of Neurological Surgeons
http://www.aans.org/en/Patient%20Information/Conditions%20and%20Treatments/Occiptal%20Neuralgia.aspx

The Trigeminal Neuralgia Association of Canada
http://tnac.org/tnac

Trigeminal Neuralgia and Hemifacial Spasm Center
neurosurgery.mgh.harvard.edu/TNHFS

The American Migraine Foundation
americanmigrainefoundation.org/about-migraine

Characteristics and causes of trigeminal neuralgia from University of Manitoba
umanitoba.ca/cranial_nerves/trigeminal_neuralgia/manuscript/types.html

Association between trigeminal neuralgia and multiple sclerosis
ncbi.nlm.nih.gov/pmc/articles/PMC486023

Trigeminal neuralgia diagnostic questionnaire from Oregon Health & Science University
https://neurosurgery.ohsu.edu/tgn.php

Striking Back: The Trigeminal Neuralgia and Face Pain Handbook
amazon.com/Striking-Back-Trigeminal-Neuralgia-Handbook/dp/096723932X

Home remedies for trigeminal neuralgia
livestrong.com/article/181886-home-remedies-for-trigeminal-neuralgia

The Patient's Journey through Trigeminal Neuralgia
iasp-pain.org/PublicationsNews/NewsletterIssue.aspx?ItemNumber=3417

Severe Facial Pain as a Symptom of Multiple Sclerosis
ms.about.com/od/signssymptoms/a/trigeminal_neur.htm

Sign the Petition!
We're asking the World Health Organization to take action on trigeminal neuralgia and facial pain disorders! To sign the petition, visit iPetitions.com/petition/trigeminal-neuralgia-awareness-day

Colorado Trigeminal Neuralgia Clinic
southdenverneurosurgery.org/home/trigeminal-neuralgia